WHY PSYCHOANALYSIS?

EUROPEAN PERSPECTIVES

A Series in Social Thought and Cultural Criticism

Lawrence D. Kritzman, Editor

EUROPEAN PERSPECTIVES presents outstanding books by leading European thinkers. With both classic and contemporary works, the series aims to shape the major intellectual controversies of our day and to facilitate the tasks of historical understanding.

For a complete list of books in the series, see pages 183–84.

WHY PSYCHOANALYSIS?

Elisabeth Roudinesco

Translated by Rachel Bowlby

COLUMBIA UNIVERSITY PRESS

NEW YORK

Columbia University Press wishes to express its appreciation for assistance given by the government of France through the Ministère de la Culture in the preparation of this translation.

Columbia University Press
Publishers Since 1893
New York   Chichester, West Sussex

Library of Congress Cataloging-in-Publication Data

Roudinesco, Elisabeth, 1944–
[Pourquoi la psychanalyse? English]
Why psychoanalysis? / Elisabeth Roudinesco ; translated by Rachel Bowlby.
p.   cm. — (European perspectives)
Includes bibliographical references and index.
ISBN 0–231–12202–0
1. Psychoanalysis. I. Title. II. Series.
BF173 .R67513 2001
150.19'5 — dc21

2001032327

Casebound editions of Columbia University Press books are printed on permanent and durable acid-free paper.
Printed in the United States of America
10 9 8 7 6 5 4 3 2 1

Human creations are easily destroyed,
and science and technology, which have built them up,
can also be used for their annihilation.

—Sigmund Freud, *The Future of an Illusion*

Contents

Translator's Note

In consultation with the author, a few clarifications and small additions have been made to the text as first published in French, particularly where cross-cultural misunderstandings might arise in relation to issues of sexual politics and the place of American psychoanalysis. All translations in the text and notes are mine, unless otherwise noted.

Rachel Bowlby

⊖

Preface

This book arose out of an observation: I wondered why it was that after a hundred years' existence and unquestionable clinical results, psychoanalysis was so violently attacked today by those claiming to replace it with drug treatments, thought to be more effective on the grounds that they get to the causes of the tortures of the soul, supposedly cerebral.

Far from contesting the usefulness of these substances and disregarding the comfort they bring, I have wanted to show that they are unable to cure people of their psychical sufferings, whether these be normal or pathological. Death, the passions, sexuality, madness, the unconscious, the relation to another: it is these that mold the subjectivity of each person, and no science worthy of the name will ever exhaust the matter, fortunately.

Psychoanalysis testifies to an advance of civilization over barbarism. It restores the idea that human speech is free and that human destiny is not confined to biological being. Thus in the future it should occupy its full place, next to the other sciences, to contest the obscurantist claims seeking to reduce thought to a neuron or to equate desire with a chemical secretion.

WHY PSYCHOANALYSIS?

PART I

The Depressive Society

CHAPTER 1

The Defeat of the Subject

Nowadays, psychical suffering manifests itself in the form of depression. Depressive people, affected body and soul by this strange syndrome mixing sadness and apathy, the quest for identity, and the cult of oneself, no longer believe in the validity of any therapy. And yet, before rejecting all treatments, they seek desperately to conquer the emptiness of their desire. They thus move from psychoanalysis to psychopharmacology, and from psychotherapy to homeopathic medicine, without taking the time to reflect on the origin of their unhappiness. And indeed they no longer have the time for anything, even as the time of life and the time of leisure, the time of unemployment and the time of boredom are extended. Depressive individuals suffer all the more from the freedoms obtained because they no longer know how to use them.[1]

The more society favors emancipation by stressing the equality of everyone before the law, the more it accentuates differences. At the heart of this structure, everyone claims his or her singularity by refusing to identify with figures of universality deemed to have fallen into decay. So the era of subjectivity has given place to the era of individuality:[2] giving themselves the illusion of a freedom without constraint, an independence without desire, and a historicity without history, people of today become the opposite of subjects. Far from constructing their beings on the basis of the consciousness of

the unconscious determinations that pass through them un-
awares, far from being biological individuals,[3] far from wanting to be free subjects, disengaged from their roots and their
collectivity, they think themselves master of a destiny whose
significance is reduced to a normative claim. Thus they attach
themselves to networks, to groups, to collectives, to communities, without managing to affirm their true *difference*.[4]

It is certainly the nonexistence of the subject that deter-
mines not only current psychopharmacological prescriptions
but the behaviors linked to psychical suffering.[5] Each patient
is treated as an anonymous being belonging to an organic totality. Immersed in a mass where each is in the image of a
clone, they find they are prescribed the same range of medications whatever their symptoms. But at the same time, they
seek another kind of outlet for their unhappiness. They fall
back on scientific medicine, and at the same time they long
for a therapy they think more appropriate to the recognition
of their identity, thereby losing themselves in the labyrinth of
alternative medicines.

Thus in Western societies we are seeing an unbelievable
growth in the little world of bonesetters, wizards, clairvoyants,
and mesmerists. In the face of a scientism elevated to the status of religion, and in the face of the cognitive sciences, which
valorize the machine-person over the desiring person,[6] we see
the counterflourishing of all sorts of practices, sometimes arising out of the prehistory of Freudianism, sometimes out of an
occult conception of body and mind: mesmerism, sophrology,
naturopathy, iridology, auriculotherapy, transpersonal ener-
getics, suggestology, mediumism, and so forth. Contrary to
what one might think, these practices attract the middle
classes—office workers, professional people, and upper-level

management—more than lower-class groups who, in spite of the increasing precariousness of social life, are still attached to a republican conception of scientific medicine.[7]

The common denominator of these practices is that they all offer a belief—and thus an illusion of cure—to people who are reasonably well off but destabilized by the economic crisis and who feel they are victims, sometimes of medical technology that is too remote from their suffering and sometimes of medicine's real inability to cure particular functional disorders. Thus the weekly news magazine *L'Express* published an opinion poll revealing that 25 percent of French people now seek a solution to their existential problems in reincarnation and the belief in previous lives.[8]

Modern democratic society wants to banish from view the reality of unhappiness, death, and violence, even as it seeks to integrate differences and resistances into a single system. It has tried to abolish the idea of social conflict, in the name of global politics and economic success. In the same way, it tends to treat revolutions as criminal and to deheroicize war, with a view to replacing politics with ethics, historical judgment with judicial sanction. It has thus moved from the age of confrontation to the age of avoidance and from the cult of glory to the valorization of the cowardly. It is not shocking nowadays to prefer Vichy to the Resistance or to transform heroes into traitors, as recently happened with Jean Moulin or Lucie and Raymond Aubrac. Never before has the duty of remembering been so celebrated, never before has there been so much preoccupation with the Shoah and the extermination of the Jews, and yet never has the reassessment of history been so far off.

Whence a conception of norm and pathology that rests on an intangible principle: each individual has the right, and thus the duty, of no longer showing their suffering, of no longer becoming enthusiastic about the tiniest ideal, other than pacifism or humanitarian morality. As a result, hatred of the other has become devious, perverse, and all the more formidable in that it puts on the mask of devotion to the victim. If hatred of the other is first of all hatred of the self, then like all masochism it rests on the imaginary negation of otherness. So the other is always a victim, and this is the reason why intolerance is generated by the wish to set up over the other the sovereign coherence of a narcissistic self whose ideal would be to destroy it before it could even exist.[9]

Since neurobiology seems to affirm that all psychical disturbances are linked to an abnormality in the functioning of nervous cells, and since adequate medication exists, why should we worry? Today, it is no longer a question of entering into struggle with the world but of avoiding litigation by applying a strategy of normalization. So it will come as no surprise that the unhappiness that one is claiming to exorcise should make its return in an overwhelming way in the field of social and affective relations: recourse to the irrational, the cult of minor differences, valorization of emptiness and stupidity, and so on. The violence of calm[10] is often more dreadful than passing through storms.

An attenuated form of the old melancholia, depression dominates contemporary subjectivity in the way that the hysteria of the end of the nineteenth century reigned in Vienna, through Anna O., Josef Breuer's famous patient, or in Paris, with Augustine, Charcot's renowned madwoman at the Salpêtrière hospital. On the eve of the third millennium, depression has become the psychical epidemic of democratic societies, even as treatments offering every consumer an honorable solution proliferate. Of course, hysteria has not disappeared, but it is increasingly experienced and treated as a form of depression. Yet this replacement of one paradigm by another is not innocent.[11]

The substitution is in fact accompanied by a valorization of the normalizing psychological processes, to the detriment of different forms of exploration of the unconscious. Treated as depression, contemporary neurotic conflict no longer seems to derive from any psychical causality arising from the unconscious. And yet the unconscious reappears through the body, opposing a strong resistance to the disciplines and practices seeking to get rid of it. Whence the relative failure of the multiplying therapies. However much they exert themselves compassionately at the bedside of the depressive subject, they don't succeed in curing her or in grasping the true causes of her torment. All they do is to improve her state by letting her hope for better days: "Depressed people suffer all over," writes the rheumatologist Marcel Francis Kahn, "which is well known. What is less well known is that one also sees conversion syndromes as spectacular as the ones observed by Charcot and Freud. Hysteria has always given pride of place to the locomotive mechanism. We are struck to see how far it can be forgotten. How far, too, the fact of mentioning hysteria gives rise, on the part of both medical and nonmedical caregivers, to anxiety, refusal, even aggression—in regard to the patient but also to the person making the diagnosis."[12]

We know that Freud's invention of a new figure of the psyche presupposed the existence of a subject capable of internalizing prohibitions. Immersed in the unconscious and riven by a guilty conscience, this subject, given up to its instincts by the death of god, is constantly at war with itself. From this follows the Freudian conception of neurosis, centered on discord, anguish, guilt, disturbances of sexuality. It is this idea of subjectivity, so characteristic of the coming of democratic societies, themselves based on the idea of permanent confrontation between the same and the other, that is being erased from contemporary mental organization, replaced by the psychological notion of depressive personality.

Derived from neurasthenia, a notion abandoned by Freud, and from the psychasthenia described by Pierre Janet, depression is not a neurosis, or a psychosis, or a form of melancholia but a feeble entity referring to a "state" thought of in terms of "fatigue," "deficit," or "weakening of the personality." The growing success of this designation demonstrates clearly that the democratic societies of the end of the twentieth century have ceased to privilege conflict as the normative kernel of the formation of subjectivity. In other words, in place of the Freudian conception of a subject of the unconscious, conscious of his or her liberty but haunted by sex, death, and prohibition, there is the more psychological conception of a depressive individual fleeing his or her unconscious and concerned to rub out the essence of all conflict in himself.[13]

Freed from prohibitions by the equalization of rights and the leveling of conditions, the depressed person at the end of the century has inherited an addictive dependence on the world. Condemned to exhaustion by the absence of a revolutionary perspective, he or she seeks in drugs or religion, in devotion to health or the cult of the perfect body, the ideal of an impossible happiness. "For this reason," concludes Alain Ehrenberg, "the drug addict is nowadays the symbolic figure used to define the features of an antisubject. In previous ages, it was the madman who occupied this place. If depression is the history of a subject who cannot be found, addiction is nostalgia for a lost subject."[14]

Instead of fighting this imprisonment, which leads to the abolition of subjectivity, depressive liberal society is happy to pursue its logic. So nowadays consumers of tobacco, alcohol, and psychotropic drugs are assimilated to drug addicts regarded as a danger to themselves and to the group. Among these new "sick people," the nicotine addicts and the alcoholics are treated as depressives to whom you prescribe psychotropic drugs. What medications of the mind will have to be invented in the future to treat the dependence of those who have been "cured" of their alcoholism, their nicotine addiction, or another addiction (to sex, food, sport, etc.) by the replacement of one form of abuse with another?

CHAPTER 2

The Medications of the Mind

Since 1950 chemical substances—or psychotropic drugs—have changed the landscape of madness. They have emptied the mental hospitals and replaced straitjackets and shock treatments with the soft wrapping of medication.[1] Although they do not cure any mental or nervous illnesses, they have revolutionized representations of the psyche by fabricating new human beings, smooth and moodless, exhausted by avoiding passions, ashamed of not conforming to the ideal offered to them.

Prescribed as much by general practitioners as by specialists in psychopathology, psychotropic drugs have the effect of normalizing behaviors and suppressing the most painful symptoms of psychical suffering without seeking to find their meaning.

Psychotropic drugs are classified into three groups: psycholeptics, psychoanaleptics, and psychodysleptics. The first group includes hypnotic drugs, which treat sleeping difficulties; anxiolytics and tranquilizers, which suppress the signs of distress, anxiety, phobia, and various other neuroses; and finally neuroleptics (or antipsychotics), medications specifically for psychosis and all forms of chronic or acute delirium. The second group brings together stimulants and antidepressives; and the third, hallucinogenic medications, narcotics, and mood-controlling drugs.

Psychopharmacology initially brought humanity a renewal of freedom. Launched in 1952 by two French psychiatrists, Jean Delay and Pierre Deniker, neuroleptics let the insane speak again. They made it possible for them to be reintegrated into society. Thanks to these drugs, barbaric and ineffective treatments were abandoned. Meanwhile, anxiolytics and antidepressants brought greater tranquility to neurotic and depressed people.

Through belief in the power of its potions, however, psychopharmacology ended up losing a part of its prestige, in spite of its formidable efficacy. In effect, what it did was to shut subjects up in a new form of alienation by claiming to cure them of the very essence of the human condition. It thereby fostered, through its illusions, a new form of irrationalism. For the more an "end" to psychical suffering is promised through the absorption of pills, which never do more than alleviate symptoms or alter a personality, the more subjects then turn, in their disappointment, to bodily or magical types of treatment.

It will come as no surprise that the excesses of pharmacology have been denounced by the very people who previously celebrated it and who nowadays demand that mind medicines be administered in a more rational way and in conjunction with other forms of cure: psychotherapy and psychoanalysis. This was already the opinion of Jean Delay, the principal French exponent of biological psychiatry, who was declaring in 1956: "We should recall that in psychiatry, medication is only one aspect of the treatment of a mental illness and that psychotherapy continues to be the fundamental treatment."[2]

And the drugs' inventor, Henri Laborit, has always maintained that psychopharmacology was not, as such, the solution to all the problems:

> Why is one happy to have psychotropic drugs? Because the society we live in is intolerable. People can't sleep anymore, they are distressed, they need to be tranquilized, more so in the big cities than elsewhere. I am sometimes reproached for having invented the chemical straitjacket. But what has no doubt been forgotten is the time when, as a duty doctor in the Marines, I entered the disturbed patients' wing with a revolver and two sturdy male nurses, because the patients were at breaking point in their straitjackets, sweating and shouting. . . . In the course of its evolution, humanity was forced to go through a drugs stage. Without psychotropic drugs, there might perhaps have been a revolution in human consciousness, saying: "We can't bear it any longer!" whereas we have continued to bear it thanks to psychotropic drugs. In a far-off future, pharmacology will perhaps appear less interesting, except perhaps in traumatology, and it is even possible to imagine that it might disappear.[3]

Even so, psychopharmacology has nowadays, in spite of itself, become the standard-bearer of a sort of imperialism. It makes it possible for all doctors—and particularly for general practitioners—to tackle all kinds of states of mind in the same way without knowing what treatment they require. Psychoses, neuroses, phobias, melancholias, and depressions are thus treated by psychopharmacology as so many anxious states resulting from bereavements, tempo-

rary panic attacks, or extreme nervousness owing to a difficult environment. "Psychotropic drugs have only become
what they are," writes Edouard Zarifian, "because they appeared at an opportune moment. They then became the
symbol of the triumph of science, science that explains the
irrational and cures the incurable. . . . Psychotropic drugs
symbolized the triumph of pragmatism and materialism
over the vague lucubrations of psychology and philosophy
that were trying to make sense of humanity."[4]

Such is the force of the ideology of medication that when
it claims to restore to men the attributes of their virility, it
provokes a flurry of madness. So the subject who thinks he is
impotent will take Viagra to put an end to his misery, without ever knowing the psychical causality from which his
symptom is derived, whereas, from another point of view, the
man whose member is really defective will also take the same
medication to improve his performance but without ever
grasping the organic cause from which his impotence is derived.[5] The same is true for the use of anxiolytics and antidepressants. "Normal" people who have been hit by a series of
misfortunes—the loss of a close relation, abandonment, unemployment, an accident—will find, if they are distressed or
in mourning, that they are prescribed the same medication as
others who have no dramatic events to deal with but are pre-
senting with identical problems because of their melancholic
or depressive psychical structure. "How many doctors,"
writes Edouard Zarifian, "prescribe a course of antidepressants to people who are simply sad and disillusioned and who
have a problem with getting to sleep because of anxiety!"[6]

The hysteria of the old days translated a protest against
the bourgeois order that manifested itself through women's

bodies. To this revolution that was powerless but strongly significant because of its sexual contents Freud accorded an emancipatory meaning that was beneficial to all women. A hundred years after this inaugural gesture, we are witnessing a regression. In democratic countries, it is as though there were no longer any possibility of revolution, as though the very idea of social and even intellectual subversion had become an illusion, as though the conformity and health-centeredness of the new barbarism of biopower had won out.[7] Whence the sadness of the soul and the impotence of the sexual organ; whence the paradigm of depression.[8]

Ten years after the worldwide celebration of the bicentennial of the French revolution, the revolutionary ideal appears to be fading away from discourses and representations. Could it continue to exercise the same fascination after the fall of the Berlin wall and the failure of the communist system?

If the emergence of the paradigm of depression does indicate that the acceptance of a norm has overtaken the valorization of conflict, that also means that psychoanalysis has lost some of its subversive force. After having contributed extensively, throughout the twentieth century, not only to the emancipation of women and oppressed minorities but to the invention of new forms of freedom, it has been dislodged, like hysteria, from the central position it used to occupy, both in therapeutically and clinically oriented subjects (psychiatry, psychotherapy, clinical psychology) and in the major disciplines it was thought to be invested in (psychology, psychopathology).

The paradox of this new situation is that now psychoanalysis is confused with the set of practices over which it used to exert its supremacy. Witness the general usage [in

French] of the prefix *psy*, jumbling together all the different strands to designate both the science of the mind and the therapeutic practices connected to it.

The word *psychoanalysis* made its appearance in 1896 in a text by Sigmund Freud written in French. A year before that, with his friend Josef Breuer, Freud had published his famous *Studies on Hysteria*, in which was recounted the case of a young Jewish Viennese girl suffering from a strange illness of psychical origin, where sexual fantasies were enacted through contortions of the body.[9] The patient was called Bertha Pappenheim, and her doctor, Breuer, who was treating her by what was known as the "cathartic" method, had given her the name "Anna O." The story of this patient would become a legend, for it was Anna O, in other words a woman and not a male expert, who was credited with the invention of the psychoanalytic method: a cure based on speech, a cure in which the fact of verbalizing suffering, of finding the words to say it, makes it possible if not to cure the suffering, then at least to become conscious of its origin and so to take it on.

Through the study of archives, modern historians have demonstrated that the famous Anna O. case, presented by Freud and Breuer as the prototype of the cathartic cure, did not really end with the patient's cure. Freud and Breuer decided in any case to publish the story of this woman and exhibit it as a definitive case, so as to improve their claim, against the French psychologist Pierre Janet, for priority in the discovery of the cathartic method.[10] As for Bertha Pappenheim, even if she was not cured of her symptoms, she certainly became another woman. A militant feminist, pious and rigid, she devoted her life to orphans and to the victims of anti-Semitism without ever speaking about the course of psychical treatment she had followed in her youth and that had made her into a myth.

Celebrated hagiographically by Freud's heirs, Anna O. thus returned to being Bertha in the writings of scholarly historiography. And by posthumously acquiring once more her actual identity, she rediscovered her true destiny, that of a tragic woman of the end of the nineteenth century who had given meaning to her existence by committing herself to a great cause. But Bertha still remained that legendary character whose rebellion had been welcomed by Breuer and Freud.

While women's bodies have become depressive and the old convulsive beauty of hysteria, so much admired by the surrealists, has been replaced with a trivial nosography,[11] psychoanalysis is suffering from the same symptom and seems no longer adapted to the depressive society, which prefers clinical psychology. It is on the way to becoming a discipline of the influential, a psychoanalysis for psychoanalysts. In 1998 Jean-Bertrand Pontalis noted this with bitterness: "Soon, psychoanalysis will only be of interest to an ever more restricted fringe of the population. Will there only be psychoanalysts left on the psychoanalysts' couch?"[12]

The more psychoanalytic institutions implode, the more present is psychoanalysis in the different spheres of society, and the more it serves as a point of historical reference for the clinical psychology that has nonetheless been substituted for it. The language of psychoanalysis has become an ordinary idiom, spoken by the masses as well as by the elite and at any rate by all the practitioners of the world of *psy*. There is no one left today who is ignorant of the Freudian vocabulary: fantasy, superego, desire, libido, sexuality, and so on.

Everywhere psychoanalysis reigns as master, but every-where it has to compete with pharmacology, and to the point of itself being used like a pill. In this regard, Jacques Derrida was right to stress, in a recent text, that these days psycho-analysis has been assimilated to an "out-of-date medicine consigned to the back of a pharmacy: 'It can always come in useful when there's an emergency or a shortage, but there's been an improved version since then.'"[13]

We do know, however, that medication is not in itself in-compatible with treatment through talking. At present, France is the European country with the highest consumption of psy-chotropic drugs (with the exception of neuroleptics), and, at the same time, the one where psychoanalysis is most firmly established, both medically and therapeutically (psychiatry, psychotherapy) and culturally (literature, philosophy). So if psychoanalysis is today set up in competition with psycho-pharmacology, this is also because the patients themselves, forced to endure the barbarity of biopolitics, now insist that their psychical symptoms must have an organic cause. And they often feel they are being treated as inferior when the doc-tor tries to show them another approach.[14]

As a result, antidepressants are prescribed more than any other psychotropic drugs, without it being possible to say definitely that states of depression are on the increase. It is simply that today's medicine is likewise responding to the paradigm of depression. Consequently, it treats almost all forms of psychical suffering as having to do with both anx-ious and depressive states.[15] Witness a number of studies that appeared in 1997 in the *Bulletin de l'Académie nationale de médecine*: "Now mainly prescribed by nonspecialists," writes Pierre Juillet:

antidepressants seem to be applicable to mood disorders on various levels, adequately in most cases but with three cycles: on the one hand, in spite of the undeniable progress in diagnosis and therapy achieved by our nonspecialist colleagues, they are prescribed for roughly half the depressions recorded among the general population; on the other hand, we are seeing a broadened definition of depression and its medicalization. . . . Presumably contemporary sociocultural developments are part of the reason for the increase in the number of ordinary people, happy to be known as "normal-neurotic," with a lowered tolerance threshold for the ineluctable habitual sufferings, difficulties, and trials of existence.[16]

All the sociological studies also show that the tendency of the depressive society is to destroy the essence of human resistance. Between the fear of disorder and the valorization of a competitiveness based only on material success, there are many subjects who prefer to give themselves over willingly to chemical substances rather than speak of their private sufferings. The power of medicines of the mind is thus the symptom of a modernity tending toward the abolition not only of the desire for liberty but also of the very idea of confronting that experience. Silence is therefore preferable to language, which is a source of distress and shame.

If patients' tolerance threshold has gone down and if their desire for liberty has decreased, the same is true for the doctors who prescribe anxiolytics and antidepressants. A recent inquiry published in the newspaper *Le Monde* shows that many nonspecialist French doctors, in particular those involved in emergency care, are no more healthy than their patients.[17] Anxious, unhappy, harassed by the laboratories, and unable to cure or, failing that, to listen to a psychical pain that overwhelms them every day, they seem to have no other solution apart from echoing the massive demand for psychotropic drugs. And who could blame them?

CHAPTER 3

The Soul Is Not a Thing

In this situation, it will come as no surprise that psycho-analysis is always being attacked by a technicist discourse constantly invoking its supposed experimental ineffective-ness. But what sort of ineffectiveness is this? Should we be-lieve Jacques Chirac when he stresses: "I have observed the effects of psychoanalysis, and I am not convinced in princi-ple, to the point that I wonder whether all this doesn't real-ly have much more to do with chemistry than psychology"? Or should we rather believe Georges Perec when he de-scribes his positive experience of analysis, or else Françoise Giroud when she asserts: "An analysis is hard, and it hurts. But when you are collapsing under the weight of repressed words, obligatory ways of behaving, the need to save face, when your representation of yourself becomes unbearable, the remedy is there. At least this is what I experienced, and I remain infinitely grateful to Jacques Lacan. . . . To stop feel-ing ashamed of yourself is the realization of freedom. . . . It is what a well-conducted analysis teaches those who come to it asking for help."[1]

Beginning in 1952, a large number of surveys were con-ducted in the United States to assess the soundness of psy-choanalyses and psychotherapies. The greatest difficulty lay in the choice of parameters. It was first of all necessary to test the difference between the absence and the existence of a treatment so as to be able to compare the effect of the passage of time (a spontaneous development) with the effectiveness of an analysis. It was next necessary to bring in the principle of the therapeutic alliance (suggestion, transference, etc.), so as to understand why some therapists, whatever their expertise, got on perfectly well with some patients and not at all with others. Finally, it was vital to take account of the subjectivity of the people being interrogated. Whence the idea of casting doubt on the authenticity of their testimonies and mistrusting the influence of the therapist.

In all the cases that figured, the patients never said they were cured of their symptoms but changed (up to 80 percent) by their experience of analysis. In other words, when analysis was beneficial, they experienced a sense of well-being or an improvement in their relationships with others, in their social and professional lives as well as in matters of love, emotion, and sex. In short, all these surveys demonstrated the extraordinary effectiveness of the whole group of psychotherapies. None of them, however, made it possible to prove statistically the superiority or inferiority of psychoanalysis over other modes of treatment.[2]

The great defect in these assessments is that they always depend on an experimental principle unsuited to the situation of analysis. Either they bring proof that it is sufficient for a suffering human being to consult a therapist for a certain length of time in order for their situation to improve, or they let it be understood that subjects who are being interrogated can be influenced by their therapists and thus victims of a placebo effect. So it is clearly because psychoanalysis refuses the very idea of experimentation being feasible by means of this kind of questioning that the so-called experimental assessment of therapeutic results has negligible value in psychoanalysis: it always reduces the soul to a thing.

When Freud was asked about this in 1934 by the psychologist Saul Rosenzweig, who had sent him some experimental results proving the validity of the theory of repression, he was both civil and prudent. He did not reject the idea of experimentation, but he stressed that the results obtained were both superfluous and redundant given the abundance of clinical experience already well established by psychoanalysis, and known through the numerous publications of case histories.[3] When another American psychologist suggested to him that he should "measure" libido and give his name (*freud*) to the unit of measurement, he also replied: " 'I do not understand enough of physics to express a reliable judgment in the matter. But if I am permitted to ask a favor, do not call your unit by my name.' With unfailing wit he added that he hoped to die someday with an unmeasured libido."[4]

The surveys have to be criticized for the way they were conducted. While many of them were conducted seriously, especially in the United States, they also gave rise to numerous controversies. Others look frankly ridiculous today. One can see that very often the questions asked determine the replies, as is shown by so-called experimental protocols that consist, for instance, in asking children aged from three to nine whether, yes or no, they are hostile to the parent of the opposite sex. It goes without saying that under these kinds of conditions, practically all the children reply that they find their parents "very nice."[5]

Psychoanalysis seems to be even more subject to attack today, when it has conquered the world through the singularity of a subjective experience that puts the unconscious, death, and sexuality at the heart of the human soul. In France, we have stopped keeping count of the press features drawing on the language of the neurosciences, cognitivism, or genetics, whose sole purpose is to wage war on Freudian thought. Up to 1995 the headings were fairly neutral and referred to a current political topic or to practical questions: "Special Freud issue: Marxism is collapsing, psychoanalysis is resisting"; or again "Do you need to be psychoanalyzed?"[6] After this, the tone became clearly anti-Freudian: "Freud: Genius or impostor?"[7] "Must we burn Lacan?" "Science against Freud."[8]

And yet, when we read the details of the interventions brought together under these catchphrases, we realize that they are saying something quite different. The reports tend to quote the words of specialists of every kind (psychologists, psychoanalysts, psychiatrists, psychotherapists, neurologists, neurobiologists, intellectuals, etc.), and a dialogue gets going—certainly in a pretty simplistic way some of the time (for or against Freud and psychoanalysis) but also, and very often, with a critical perspective and with respect for the different disciplines. Most of the time, the men of science manifest prudence. Apart from a few who are inflexible, the researchers questioned never wish to burn anyone at all.

Why, nonetheless, does psychoanalysis arouse such strong disapproval? What has happened for it to be both so present in debates about the future of humanity and so unattractive in the eyes of those who see it as old, out of fashion, ineffective?[9] The meaning of this discredit must be sought in the recent transformation of the models of thinking developed by dynamic psychiatry. The perception of the status of madness in Western societies has been based on these for the past two centuries.

The term *dynamic psychiatry* refers to the group of tendencies and schools linking a description of the illnesses of the soul (madness), the nerves (neurosis), and mood (melancholia) with a psychical treatment of a dynamic nature, in other words, bringing in a transferential relationship between the doctor and the patient.[10] Derived from medicine, dynamic psychiatry privileges psychogenesis (psychical causality) over organogenesis (organic causality) without, however, ruling the latter out, and it is based on four major explanatory models for the human psyche: a nosographic model arising from psychiatry and enabling both a universal classification of illnesses and a definition of clinical practice in terms of norms and pathology; a psychotherapeutic model inherited from the ancient healers and assuming that therapeutic efficacy is linked to a power of suggestion; a philosophical or phenomenological model making it possible to grasp the meaning of the psychical or mental trouble starting from what is lived and existential (both consciously and unconsciously) for the subject; and a cultural model proposing to discover in the diversity of mentalities, societies, and religions an anthropological explanation of humanity based on social context or difference.

In general, schools and tendencies have privileged one or two models of interpretation of the psyche, varying with countries or periods. Psychiatric knowledge has mainly been organized through the association of a rational classification of mental illnesses with a "moral treatment" [see below], but the various schools of psychotherapy, on the other hand, have sometimes favored a relational technique from which nosography was excluded, sometimes a form of ethnopsychology taking patients, and humanity in general, back to their roots, their ghettos, their communities or origins.[11]

Originating with Philippe Pinel, the nosological model developed throughout the nineteenth century, referring back to the famous myth of the abolition of the chains, invented under the Restoration by the son of the founding father and his principal pupil, Etienne Esquirol. What is this about? Under the Terror, shortly after being appointed to Bicêtre hospital (September 11, 1793), Pinel received a visit from Couthon, a member of the committee for public safety, who was looking for suspects among the insane. They all trembled before this loyal servant of Robespierre, who had left his paralytic's chair to have himself carried along supported by men's arms. Pinel led him in front of the cells where the sight of the agitated men caused him intense fear. Greeted by insults, he turned to the alienist and said: "Citizen, are you mad yourself to want to free animals like these?" The doctor replied that mad people were all the less capable of being treated because they were deprived of air and freedom. Couthon agreed that the chains should be stopped, but he put Pinel on guard against his presumption. So it was that the philanthropist began his life's work: he unleashed the insane and thereby gave birth to alienism and then to psychiatry.[12]

Pinel's revolution consisted in ceasing to regard the mad person as someone senseless, whose speech was devoid of sense, but rather as someone alienated, in other words, as a subject strange to himself; not an animal put in a cage and stripped of his humanity on the grounds that he is deprived of reason but a human being recognized as such. The nosographic model, which comes from alienism, organizes the human psyche on the basis of large meaningful structures (psychoses, neuroses, perversions, phobia, hysteria, etc.) that define the principle of a norm and a pathology and set the boundaries between reason and unreason.[13] This model is closely linked to that of psychotherapy, whose origin goes back to Franz Anton Mesmer. A man of the Enlightenment, Mesmer sought to wrest the obscure part of the human soul away from religion. His ideas were based on the false theory of animal magnetism, which was to be abandoned by his successors. He treated hysterics and possessed women without the help of magic, using only the force of a power of suggestion. Pinel's contribution, shortly after the Revolution, was the invention of the "moral treatment" at the same time as William Tuke, the English Quaker.

He reformed clinical practice by showing that there always subsists a remainder of reason in the insane patient, which makes possible the therapeutic relationship. Separated from other forms of unreason (vagrancy, begging, deviance), madness, as defined by Pinel, became an illness. From then on, people who were mad could be looked after with the help of an adequate nosography and an appropriate treatment. Asylums—and later psychiatric hospitals—were invented for them, so as to distance them from the general Hospital, that symbol of imprisonment in the European monarchies. Then Esquirol gave Pinel's teaching a doctrinal content that resulted, in 1838, in the asylum system being made official.

Between mesmerism and the Pinel revolution, the first dynamic psychiatry associated a nosographic model (psychiatry) with a psychotherapeutic model (magnetism, suggestion) that separated the madness of asylums (illnesses of the soul, psychoses) from ordinary madness (illnesses of the nerves, neuroses). A century later, Jean-Martin Charcot, its last great representative, annexed neurosis (that semimadness) to the nosographic model by making it into a functional disorder. But the asylum nonetheless remained dominant, with its train of distresses, cries, and cruelties. Having attained great sophistication, psychiatry at the end of the nineteenth century lost interest in the subject, abandoning him or her to barbaric treatments in which speech had no place. Preferring to classify illnesses rather than listen to suffering, it sank into a kind of therapeutic nihilism.

Successor to Charcot, the second dynamic psychiatry derived its impetus from a loud affirmation of the founding gesture of Pinel. Without giving up the nosographic model, it reinvented a psychotherapeutic model by letting the ill person speak, as did Hippolyte Bernheim in Nancy and, later, Eugen Bleuler in Zurich. It then found its completed form in the modern schools of psychology (Freud and Janet). Against the grain of this movement, what we are seeing today is the dislocation of the four major models and the rupture of the balance that made it possible to organize their diversity.

Confronted by the growth of psychopharmacology, psychiatry has let go of the nosographic model in favor of a classification of forms of behavior. As a result, it has reduced psychotherapy to a technique for eradicating symptoms. Whence an empirical and nontheoretical valorization of emergency treatments. Whatever the length of the prescription, the medicine is always a response to a crisis situation, a symptomatic state. Whether the problem is one of distress, agitation, melancholy, or straightforward anxiety, it will first be necessary to treat its visible trace, then to eradicate it, and finally to avoid seeking out its cause, in such a way as to orient the patient toward a less and less conflictual and thus more and more depressive position. Calm in place of the passions, absence of desire in place of desire, nothingness in place of the subject, the end of history in place of history. Modern caregivers—psychologists, psychiatrists, nurses, or doctors—no longer have time to concern themselves with the long term of the psyche because, in depressive liberal society, their time is limited.

CHAPTER 4

Behavior-Modification Man

Depressive society, written into the movement of economic globalization that is transforming people into objects, no longer wants to hear talk of guilt, or of personal meaning, or of conscience, or of desire, or of unconscious. The more it imprisons itself in narcissistic logic, the more it is running away from the idea of subjectivity. So depressive society is only interested in the individual for the purpose of calculating his or her successes and only interested in the suffering subject for the purpose of regarding him or her as a victim. And if depressive society is always seeking to put the deficit into figures, to measure the handicap, quantify the degree of trauma, this is so that it will never again have to ask itself questions about their origin.

The sick person in depressive society is thus literally possessed by a biopolitical system that governs his or her thinking like a great sorcerer. Not only is he not responsible for anything in his life, but he no longer has the right to imagine that his death could be an act that depends on his consciousness or unconscious. Recently, for instance, without there being the slightest proof and despite lively protestations on the part of numerous psychiatrists, an American researcher claimed that the exclusive cause of suicide lay not in in a subjective decision, a taking of action, or a historical context but in an abnormal production of serotonin.[1] This, in the name of a purely chemico-biological logic, would be the effacement of the tragic nature of a fundamentally human act: from Cleopatra to Cato of Utica, from Socrates to Mishima, from Werther to Emma Bovary. It would also mean, by virtue of a mere molecule, the wiping out of all the sociological, historical, philosophical, literary, and psychoanalytical studies, from Emile Durkheim to Maurice Pinguet, that have given ethical, not chemical, significance to the long tragedy of voluntary death.[2]

It is through the adoption of identical principles that some geneticists claim to explain the origin of most forms of human behavior. Since 1990 they have been attempting to bring into play what they call the genetic mechanisms of homosexuality, social violence, alcoholism, or schizophrenia.

In 1991 Simon LeVay claimed to have discovered the secret of homosexuality in the hypothalamus. Two years later, another American expert, Dean Hamer, took this further by declaring that he, too, had isolated the homosexuality chromosome on the basis of observations of forty or so sets of male twins. Then there was Hans Brunner, a Dutch geneticist, who in 1993 had no hesitation in establishing a relationship between the abnormal behavior of different members of a family who had been accused of rape or arson and the mutation of a gene with the task of programming a brain enzyme (monamine oxydase A).

These findings were published in the journal *Science* and spread internationally in the press, even though they were violently accused of "neurogenetic reductionism" by other experts. Witness the courageous intervention of Steven Rose, the eminent British neurobiologist:

Today these ideas are becoming significant in countries such as the United States or Great Britain because their deeply right-wing governments are desperately seeking to find individual solutions to social problems. . . . After Dean Hamer's article on gay genes, numerous critiques appeared, and as yet his data have not been reproduced either by himself or by anyone else. . . . Generally speaking, it is interesting to note that some scientific journals publish research on human beings that is so bad it would have been rejected if it had been on animals. . . . All this research is a result of the catastrophic loss that has affected the Western world in the last few years. Loss of hope of finding social solutions to social problems. Disappearance of socialist democracies and, for some, of the belief that there was a better society in Eastern Europe. . . . Recently, as a joke, I wrote in the journal *Nature* that with this type of research someone would soon be claiming that the war in Bosnia was the result of a serotonin problem in Dr. Karadzic's brain and that it could be stopped by a massive prescription of Prozac.[3]

The consequence of the systematic recourse to the vicious circle of external causality—genes, neurones, hormones, and so on—has been the dislocation of dynamic psychiatry and its replacement by a behavioral system in which there are only two explanatory models: on one side, organicity, bearer of a simplistic universality; and, on the other, difference, bearer of an empirical culturalism. Whence there results a reductive split between the world of reason and the universe of mentalities, between the affections of the body and those of the mind, between the universal and the particular.

This is the split that is at the origin of the current valorization of explanation in terms of ethnicity (or identity),[4] which is coming to take the place of reference to the psychical.[5] Set apart from the other major models of dynamic psychiatry, the culturalist model can seem to involve a humanization of suffering, whereas in reality it lets patients think their suffering derives not from themselves or their relations with others but from ill-willed people, from the stars, from fortune-tellers, or, in a word, from culture and what is called ethnic belonging: an elsewhere for which another elsewhere can always be substituted. So explanation in terms of the cultural is like organic causality and sends the subject back to the universe of possession.

At the end of his life, Freud was aware that the progress of pharmacology would one day impose limits on the technique of the talking cure: "The future may teach us to exercise a direct influence, by means of particular chemical substances, on the amounts of energy and their distribution in the mental apparatus. It may be that there are other still undreamt-of possibilities of therapy. But for the moment we have nothing better at our disposal than the technique of psycho-analysis, and, for that reason, in spite of its limitations, it should not be despised."[6]

While Freud was not wrong, he was a long way from imagining that psychiatric knowledge would be destroyed by psychopharmacology. And he did not imagine that the extension of psychoanalytic practice to most Western countries would occur at the same time as this progressive destruction and the deployment of chemical substances in the treatment of the maladies of the soul. For not only is the *pharmakon* not in opposition to the psychical, but the two have historically been in alliance, as Gladys Swain stresses very well: "The point at which the whole panoply of neuroleptics and antidepressants gets deployed on a vast scale in psychiatric practice and transforms it is also the point at which a psychoanalytic orientation and the institutional option become dominant in it."[7]

In principle, it ought to have been possible to maintain a balance between treatment with psychotropic drugs and psychoanalysis, between the evolution of the sciences of the brain and the perfecting of explanations of the psyche through models of meaning making. But this was not the case. Beginning in the 1980s, all the rational psychical treatments inspired by psychoanalysis were violently attacked in the name of the spectacular progress of psychopharmacology. To the point that psychiatrists themselves, as I have said, are worried about it and strongly criticize its harmful and perverse effects. What they are afraid of is seeing the disappearance of their discipline to make way for a hybrid practice. On the one hand, this would restrict hospitalization to cases of chronic madness, thought of in terms of organic illness and linked to medicine, and, on the other, patients not mad enough to be dealt with by a psychiatric knowledge entirely dominated by psychotropic drugs and the neurosciences would get referred to clinical psychologists.

To get a sense of the impact of this worldwide mutation, one has only to study the evolution of the famous *Diagnostic and Statistical Manual of Mental Disorders (DSM)*, of which the first version (*DSM I*) was put together by the American Psychiatric Association (APA) in 1952.[8]

At that time, the *Manual* took account of the findings of psychoanalysis and dynamic psychiatry. It defended the idea that psychical and mental disorders essentially derived from the subject's unconscious history, place in the family, and relationship to the social environment. In other words, it blended a triple approach: the cultural (or social), the existential, and the pathological correlated to a norm. In this view of things, the notion of organic causality was not disregarded, and psychopharmacology, which was rapidly expanding, was utilized in association with the talking cure or other dynamic therapies.

But with the development of a free-market approach to treatments, subjecting clinical practice to a criterion of profitability, the Freudian hypotheses were judged to be inefficient for therapeutic purposes: it was said that the cure was too long and too costly. Plus the fact that its results could not be measured: when you asked people who had been in analysis about it, didn't they generally reply that they had been changed by their experience, but that even so they couldn't call themselves cured?

The nuance is fitting, and it touches on the very definition of the status of the cure in psychoanalysis. In fact, as I have mentioned, in the field of the psychical there is no cure in the sense that is meant in that of somatic illnesses, genetic or organic. In scientific medicine, effectiveness rests on the model signs-diagnosis-treatment. You observe symptoms (fever), you name the illness (typhoid), you administer a treatment (antibiotics). The sick person is then cured from the biological mechanism of the illness.[9] In other words, unlike traditional forms of medicine, for which soul and body form a totality included in a cosmogony, scientific medicine rests on a separation between these two domains. Where the psychical is concerned, however, the symptoms do not refer back to a single illness, and nor is this exactly an illness (in the somatic sense) but a state. So a cure is nothing other than an existential transformation of the subject.

After 1952 the *Manual* was revised a number of times by the APA, tending toward a radical abandonment of the synthesis achieved by dynamic psychiatry. Modeled on the sign-diagnosis-treatment schema, it ended up eliminating subjectivity itself from its classifications. Four revisions took place: 1968 (*DSM II*), 1980 (*DSM III*), 1987 (*DSM III-R*), and 1994 (*DSM IV*). The result of this progressive cleaning-up operation, called "theoretical," was a disaster. Its fundamental aim was to demonstrate that any disturbances of the soul and the psyche had to be reduced to the equivalent of a motor breakdown.

Whence the elimination of all the terminology developed by psychiatry and psychoanalysis. Concepts (psychosis, neurosis, perversion) were replaced by the soft notion of "disorder," and clinical entities abandoned in favor of a symptomatic characterization of these vaunted disorders. So hysteria was reduced to being a disorder of dissociation, or "conversion," liable for treatment as a depressive illness; and schizophrenia was assimilated to a disturbance of the course of thinking; and so on.

Seeking, moreover, to avoid all controversy, the different versions of the *DSM* ended up abolishing the very idea of illness. The expression "mental disorder" served to bypass the delicate problem of the inferiorization of patients. If they were treated as ill, there was a risk of their demanding "reparation" from *DSM* practitioners and even of their taking them to court. The same kind of thinking led to the replacement of the adjective "alcoholic" by "alcohol-dependent," and it was deemed preferable to give up the notion of "schizophrenia" for a periphrasis: "affected by disorders deriving from a disturbance of a schizophrenic type."

Equally concerned to preserve cultural differences, the authors of the *DSM* discussed the question of whether so-called deviant political, religious, or sexual forms of conduct should or should not be regarded as behavioral disorders. They concluded in the negative but also affirmed that the "agnostic" criterion only made sense if patients belonged to an ethnic group different from that of the person examining them.[10]

Along with each of the different revisions, the *DSM*'s promoters sunk themselves a little deeper into the ridiculous. Between 1973 and 1975 they even came to forget the fundamental principles of science.

For "homosexuality," they substituted "ego-dystonic homosexuality," the expression designating those whose drives plunge them into depression. As Lawrence Hartmann pointed out, it was thus very much a matter of eliminating a whole nosography so as to replace it by the description of a depressive or anxious state capable of being treated by by psychopharmacology or behavior modification therapy: "I find it preferable not to use the word homosexual, which can be harmful to people. The word *depression* is not a problem, nor is *anxiety neurosis*. . . . I use the vaguest and most general categories provided that they are compatible with my concern for truth. Insurance companies are well aware that the diagnostic labels communicated to them are toned down so as not to disadvantage patients."[11]

In 1975 a committee of black psychiatrists demanded the inclusion of racism among mental disorders. Robert Spitzer, the chief editor of the *Manual*, rightly refused this suggestion, though he gave a nonsensical definition of racism: "In the context of *DSM III*, we should cite racism as a good example of a state corresponding to a non-optimal mode of psychological functioning which, in certain circumstances, renders the person fragile and leads to the appearance of symptoms."[12]

The principles articulated in the *Manual* carry authority the world over since their adoption by the World Psychiatric Association (WPA), founded in 1950 by Henri Ey, and then by the World Health Organization (WHO). In the tenth revision of its classification of illnesses (CIM-10), in chapter F, the WHO in fact defines mental disorders and behavioral disorders according to the same criteria as those of *DSM IV*. Finally, after 1994, in the new revision of the *DSM* (or *DSM IV-R*), the same principles—called *zero-to-three* (or 0–3)—have been added to the study of behaviors in babies and very young children deemed dissociative, traumatic, and depressive.

The dislocation of the four great models, which had allowed dynamic psychiatry to link a theory of the subject to a nosology and an anthropology, thus had the effect of separating psychoanalysis from psychiatry, of bringing psychiatry back into the field of a bio-physiological medicine excluding subjectivity, and then of favoring a formidable explosion of claims to identity and psychotherapeutic schools, first in the United States and then in every European country.

These psychotherapeutic schools arose at the same time as psychoanalysis; what they have in common is that they all bypass the three Freudian concepts of the unconscious, sexuality, and the transference. They oppose a cerebral, biological, or automatic subconscious to the Freudian unconscious; instead of sexuality in the Freudian sense, they prefer sometimes a culturalist theory of the difference of the sexes or races and sometimes a theory of instincts. Finally, they oppose a therapeutic relationship derived from suggestion to the idea of the transference as the driving force of the clinical practice of analysis.

So almost all these schools offer subjects, saturated as they are with medications, external causations, astrology, and *DSM*, a more humanist therapeutic relationship, better adapted to their demands. And probably, in this kind of context, it is inevitable and even necessary that psychotherapies should move on. In other words, if the nineteenth century was indeed the century of psychiatry, and if the twentieth was the century of psychoanalysis, then we may wonder whether the next one won't be the century of psychotherapies.

Yet we do have to recognize that only psychoanalysis has been able, ever since its beginnings, to bring about the synthesis of the four great models of dynamic psychiatry that are necessary for the rational apprehension of madness and psychical illness. What it did was to borrow psychiatry's nosographic model, psychotherapy's model of psychical treatment, philosophy's theory of the subject, and anthropology's conception of culture based on the idea of a universality of the human race respectful of differences.

Thus psychoanalysis cannot as such contribute to the currently dominant idea of the reduction of the psychical organization to forms of behavior without disgracing itself. If the term *subject* has meaning, subjectivity is neither measurable nor quantifiable: it is the conscious and unconscious test, both visible and invisible, by which the essence of human experience is affirmed.

⊖

PART II

The Great Quarrel Over the Unconscious

CHAPTER 5

Frankenstein's Brain

In December 1980, in a famous lecture, "The Brain and Thought," Georges Canguilhem reaffirmed the hostility he had expressed toward psychology in 1956, accusing it of relying on biology and physiology to maintain that thinking is only the effect of a secretion from the brain.[1] In this lecture, psychology is no longer designated just as "a philosophy without rigor," an "ethics that makes no demands," and a "medicine with no control";[2] it is assimilated to sheer barbarism.

Without using the word *cognitivism*, which was to appear in 1981, Canguilhem makes a ferocious attack on the belief that animates the cognitive ideal: claiming to want to create a science of the mind based on a correlation between mental states and states of the brain. He is clearly referring to the work of Alan Turing, Norbert Wiener, and Noam Chomsky, and he severely criticizes the imperialism of these doctrines that, since the time of phrenology, have been contributing, whatever their differences, to the growth of this science of the mind:

Briefly: before phrenology, Descartes was thought of as a thinker, an author responsible for his philosophical system. According to phrenology, Descartes is the bearer of a brain that thinks under the name of René Descartes. . . . In short, starting from the image of Descartes's brain, the learned phrenologist concludes that all of Descartes, biography and philosophy, is in a brain that we have to call *his* brain, Descartes's brain, since the brain contains the faculty of perceiving the actions that are in him. But finally *what* him? This is where we reach the heart of the ambiguity. Who or what says *I*?[3]

Not content with thrashing all those who want to discover the seat of thought in an image of the brain, Canguilhem stresses how ridiculous it is to declare, as do the theorists of artificial intelligence, that there is an analogy between the brain and the computer and that this justifies making the production of thought the equivalent of a flow, as in the science of robotics:

> What is now the stale metaphor of the computer-brain is justified to the extent that what we mean by thought is logical operations, calculation, reasoning. . . . But whether we are considering analogical machines or logic, calculation or data processing according to instructions is one thing, the invention of a theorem quite another. Calculating a rocket's path is for computers. Formulating the law of universal attraction is a performance that is not for computers. No invention [is] without a logical void, without a striving toward a possibility, without the risk of being wrong.   (p. 21)

And Canguilhem adds: "I have deliberately chosen not to deal with a question that logically ought to lead us to wonder about the possibility of one day seeing in a bookstore window *The Autobiography of a Computer*, without its *Autocritique*

[Self-Critique]" (p. 24).[4] Ultimately, Canguilhem is simply sending those he criticizes back to Claude Bernard's famous pronouncement: "A skillful hand without the head that directs it is a blind instrument: the head without the fulfilling hand remains powerless."[5]

If the brain cannot be assimilated to a machine, and if it is not possible to give an account of thought without reference to a conscious subjectivity, it is also impossible, says Canguilhem, to reduce mental functioning to a chemical activity. It is stating the obvious to say that there would be no thought without cerebral activity, but it is contrary to the truth to claim that the brain produces thought only as a result of its chemical activity: "Consequently, despite the existence and the fortunate effects of certain chemical mediators, despite the perspectives opened up by certain discoveries in neuro-endocrinology, the time does not yet appear ripe to announce in Cabanis's style that the brain is going to secrete thought as the liver secretes bile" (p. 23).

In this lecture, Canguilhem does not concern himself with the quarrels between behaviorists and cognitivists, between neurobiologists and physicalists. He makes a general attack on an eclectic approach in which behaviorism, experimentalism, cognitive science, artificial intelligence, and so forth are mixed, not on the sciences and their advances, not on modern work on neurones, genes, or cerebral activity. In short, in Canguilhem's eyes, this psychology that claims to take its models from science is just an instrument of power, a biotechnology of human behavior, stripping humanity of its subjectivity and seeking to take away its freedom of thought.[6]

In order to fight this psychology, Canguilhem uses Freud to support his case. He shows that the Viennese pioneer was the only scholar of his time to have theorized the hypothesis of the existence of the psyche starting from the notion of a psychical apparatus. Between 1895, the year he wrote his *Project for a Scientific Psychology*, and 1915, the date when he elaborated his metapsychology, Freud takes note of the failure of contemporary projects that tend to make psychical processes dependent on the organization of the nerve cells. He thus takes his distance more firmly than ever from the idea of a resemblance between a topical organization of the unconscious and an anatomy of the brain.

I have quoted Georges Canguilhem's lecture at length because it seems to me an exemplary illustration of the great quarrel that for over a century has set partisans of a possible constitution of a science of the mind, with the mental modeled on the neural, against supporters of an autonomy of the psychical processes. At the center of this dispute, the Freudian unconscious becomes the object of a particular controversy to the extent that its definition escapes the categories belonging to either domain. Not only is this unconscious not assimilable to a neural system, but it cannot be integrated with a cognitive or experimental conception of psychology. And yet it doesn't belong to the domain of the occult or the irrational. In other words, in relation to other definitions of the unconscious, the Freudian unconscious initially emerges negatively: it is neither hereditary, nor cerebral, nor automatic, nor neural, nor cognitive, nor metaphysical, nor metapsychical, nor symbolic, and so on. But then what is its nature, and why is it constantly the point at issue for bitter polemics?

Canguilhem's lecture is exemplary for another reason. What it shows is that it is almost always the most positivist scholars, the ones most firmly attached to the principles of hard-core science, who elaborate the most extravagant and irrational theories of the brain and the psyche, once they claim to be applying their results to the whole set of human processes. The quest for total rationalization, which basically seeks to master the fabrication of humans, is only a new version of the myth of Prometheus.

In the modern period, it is Mary Shelley who has given the finest expression of this, in a famous novel published in 1817: *Frankenstein; or, The Modern Prometheus*. In it, she tells the story of a young scholar, Victor Frankenstein, who decides to fabricate a human being without a soul by putting together pieces of corpses taken from cemeteries or mortuaries. But once he has been created, the monster becomes humanized and suffers from being deprived of the divine spark that is the only thing that would enable him to live. So he asks his creator to make him a woman in his own image. After some dreadful arguments, the monster disappears into the frozen desert of the Arctic after killing the scientist. As Mary Shelley gave the creature no name, successive readers and commentators have confused it with the scientist himself. This is how Frankenstein, this unnameable and tragic thing, has come to testify to a great nightmare of Western reason.[7]

The project of extending scientific discourse to the full range of human phenomena was established between 1870 and 1880, influenced by Darwinian evolutionary theory. Whence the spread of all -*ism* terms assumed to bring a scientific legitimacy to rational forms of knowledge as well as to questionable doctrines inspired by science.

As a lay theology,[8] scientism constantly accompanied the discourse of science and the evolution of sciences (in the plural), claiming to resolve all human problems through a belief in the absolute determination of Science's capacity to resolve them. In other words, scientism is a religion in the same way as those it wants to combat. It is an illusion of science in the sense that Freud defines religion as an illusion.[9] But, much more than a religion, the scientistic illusion claims to make up for all the uncertainties that are necessary to the deployment of a scientific investigation, through mythologies or crazy fantasies.

If scientific discourse is capable of appropriating Frankenstein's brain to make it into an emblem of a modern rationality, it will come as no surprise that some of the best contemporary specialists in cerebral biology can fall into the same trap and, as a result, come to denounce psychoanalysis as a mythological, literary, or shamanistic doctrine.

How, for instance, is it possible to take seriously the declarations of Henri Korn, a French neurobiologist, when he asserts that psychoanalysis is just a "shamanism without a theory"?[10] How can we contain ourselves at the proclamations of Jean-Pierre Changeux, a professor at the Collège de France, when he claims to reduce all forms of thought to a "cerebral machine" and declares, contrary to the doctors themselves, that he supports the wholesale adoption of a biological psychiatry based on the primacy of pharmacology and freed from "the imperialism of psychoanalytic discourse" or "Freudian mythologies" professed by "a certain Left Bank café culture"?[11] And how should we understand the declarations of the French philosopher Marcel Gauchet when he claims to put the cerebral unconscious and the model of the computer in place of the Freudian unconscious, which apparently no longer "pays" in a world in which "affect" is on the way out?[12]

And how, finally, can we accept the predictions of the American political scientist Francis Fukuyama when he congratulates himself on the "disappearance" of psychoanalysis, history, and the whole set of "constructed" theories, which have made way for the coming of a society based on natural science, one that has abolished humanity itself? "At this point," he writes, "we will have definitively finished with human history because we will have abolished human beings as such. Then a new history will begin, beyond the human."[13]

Of course, these excesses are denounced by other scholars who do not hesitate to castigate the scientistic illusions of their colleagues. So Gerald Edelman, American neurologist and winner of the Nobel prize for medicine, maintains that the unconscious, in the Freudian sense, remains an indispensable notion for the scientific understanding of human mental life. In a work entitled *The Remembered Present: A Theory of the Biology of Consciousness*, he further shows that hostility to the Freudian model derives not so much from scientific discussion as from the resistance of the scholars themselves to their own unconsciouses:

> With my late friend Jacques Monod, a great molecular biologist, I often had heated discussions about Freud. He stubbornly maintained that Freud was anti-scientific and probably a charlatan. On my side, I defended the idea that, while he wasn't scientific in our sense of the term, Freud had been a great pioneer intellectual, particularly with regard to his vision of the unconscious and its role in behavior. Monod's response to that—he came from a strict Protestant family—would be: "I am completely conscious of my motivations and entirely responsible for my

actions. They are all conscious." In exasperation, I once retorted: "Jacques, let's just say that everything Freud said applies to me and none of it applies to you." "Exactly, dear friend," he replied.[14]

Like Edelman, the French neurobiologist Alain Prochiantz stresses that for him, and contrary to Jean-Pierre Changeux, no contradiction exists between the science of the brain, genetics, and psychoanalytic doctrine: "If genes define our belonging to the species and our physical type, they do not on their own determine our personalities as thinking beings. The brain is not a computer with its codes dictated by the genetic apparatus."[15]

Freud was closely attached to the most developed science of his time and wanted to make psychology into a natural science. This is why, in an incomplete manuscript that he wrote at fever pitch in 1895,[16] he posited a certain number of correlations between the structures of the brain and the psychical apparatus, by trying to represent psychical processes as so many quantitative states determined by material particles or "neurones." He classified these into three distinct systems: perception (phi neurones), memory (psi neurones), and consciousness (omega neurones). As to the energy transmitted (quantity), it was governed, Freud thought, by two principles—one of inertia, the other of constancy—and it derived either from the external world, and so was carried by the sense organs, or from the internal world (meaning the body). Freud's ambition at this time was certainly to bring everything in normal or pathological psychical functioning back to this neurophysiological model: desire, hallucinatory states, ego functions, the mechanism of the dream, and so forth.

This need to "neurologize" the psychical apparatus in fact, as Henri F. Ellenberger stresses, amounted to an obedience to a scientistic representation of physiology and a fabrication, once again, of a "cerebral mythology."[17] Freud became aware of this and gave up this project in order to construct a purely psychological theory of the unconscious. Nonetheless, even if he was declaring in 1915 that "every attempt to . . . discover a localisation of mental processes, every endeavor to think of ideas as stored up in nerve-cells and of excitations as travelling along nerve-fibres, has miscarried completely," he never abandoned the idea that a localization of this kind might one day be demonstrated: "The deficiencies in our description would probably vanish if we were already in a position to replace the psychological terms by physiological or chemical ones."[18]

Since its posthumous publication in 1950, the *Project for a Scientific Psychology* has been the subject of countless commentaries and caused a lot of ink to flow.[19] For classical Freudians, this manuscript merely represents a stage in the construction of a true theory of the unconscious, freed from any cerebral substratum. And if Freud rejected the text to the extent that he never claimed it back from his friend Wilhelm Fliess, that certainly indicates that he was always haunted, even in abandoning it, by the temptation to "naturalize" the science of the mind. So the *Project* has remained a sort of invisible ghost, forever passing across all his writings.

For the adversaries of psychoanalysis, the publication of this manuscript was a gift. It gave them the right to declare that Freud had definitively departed from the domain of true (so-called natural) science, choosing the path of what they called "nonscience," meaning the irrational, literature, mythology, the "nonrefutable." There was thus no longer any need to discuss his conception of the unconscious, since psychoanalysis no longer derived from any possible scientific evaluation.

In reality, hostility to Freudian theses had begun well before the contents of the *Project* became known.

Scholarly historiography has shown that Freud was in fact neither the inventor of the word *unconscious* nor the first to discover its existence.[20] As far back as classical times, questions were already being asked about the idea of a psychical activity involving something other than consciousness. Descartes, however, was the first to posit the principle of a dualism of body and mind. That led him to make the cogito the seat of reason, as opposed to the universe of unreason. Unconscious thought was thereby domesticated, to be either annexed to reason or rejected into madness.[21]

Early dynamic psychiatry was based on the idea that consciousness was threatened by forces that were unknown, dangerous, and destructive, localized in a metapsychical (or subliminal) unconscious that could be reached through spiritual methods, meaning via the words of a medium capable of communicating with the dead by making tables go round. It was within this framework, explored by the treatments based on magnetism, that the unconscious then came to be regarded not as an occult force come from the beyond but as a dissociation of consciousness. At this time it was described in terms of subconscious, supraconscious, or automatism (mental or psychological), attainable through hypnosis (Charcot) or by suggestion (Hippolyte Bernheim), meaning through sleep or personal influence. Adopted at the end of the nineteenth century by most schools of psychology, as well as by psychotherapists, this unconscious accounted rationally for all the phenomena of double consciousness, somnambulism, and multiple personalities. This is how there came to be a project of observing, describing, or caring for disturbances of identity manifested by the coexistence in a single subject of a number of personalities, separated from one another and able to get him or her to live multiple lives.

In the same period, the different theories of heredity, borrowed from Darwinism and evolutionism, gave birth to a conception of the unconscious adapted to the principles of racial psychology. This hereditary unconscious, collective and individual, was thought to be molded from traces or stigmata that determined a subject's membership of a race, an ethnic group, an archetype, or even a pathology thought of in terms of degeneration. This conception can be found in numerous areas of knowledge at the end of the nineteenth century: from the sexological theories of Richard von Krafft-Ebing, who treated the sexual perversions as defects, to Cesare Lombroso's theses on the born criminal, or those of Gustave Le Bon, which assimilate crowds to damaging, hysterical masses, or again those of Georges Vacher de Lapouge, advocating the necessity of eugenics.

The emergence of this theory of a hereditary unconscious was perfectly described by Michel Foucault in *The Will to Knowledge*.[22] Coming at the same time as the end of the belief in social privilege, it cultivates the bourgeois ideal of "good race" and depends on anti-Semitism, antiegalitarianism, and hatred of crowds and people on the margins, proposing a new representation of the relationship between the social body, the individual body, and the "mental," conceived of as organic entities and described in terms of norm and pathology.

This conception leads to two antagonistic ideas. One takes degeneration literally and proclaims the loss of a humanity engulfed by its instincts. It results in eugenicism and genocide. Against the radical evil, the remedy has to be even more radical: on one side, selection so as to preserve the good race; on the other, extermination to make the bad one disappear.

The second route is that of a belief in good health, through the cure of one person by another. This method therefore proposes to fight the defects prophylactically, psychologically, pedagogically. In short, it sets the human sciences to work on the reeducation of souls and bodies. Against the idea of fall and decadence, it develops that of human redemption through science, knowledge, self-analysis, and introspection.

Corresponding to this hereditary unconscious is a cerebral unconscious derived from the physiology of reflexes. The notion comes from the description proposed by neurophysiologists of spinal then cerebrospinal activity, inducing cerebral changes in humans independently of consciousness and will. This conception of the unconscious, organized around the central function of memory, occurs extensively in the *Project*, as well as in the works of Théodule Ribot and Henri Bergson. It is based on the idea that the brain can act as a support for a disqualification of the classical function of consciousness.[23]

From Schelling to Nietzsche to Schopenhauer, German philosophy in the nineteenth century also worked to forge its own conception of the unconscious. In stressing the nocturnal side of the soul, it caused the emergence of the modern idea that consciousness is in some sense determined by another place of the psyche: its deep and shadowy side. All the work in physiology and experimental psychology that would inspire Freud, from Herbart to Wundt via Helmholtz and

Fechner, unfolded out of this philosophical conception of the unconscious, strongly tinted with romanticism.[24]

Freud brings about the synthesis of these different conceptions of the unconscious, but in doing this he invents a new one. For him, the unconscious is no longer either an automatic function, or a subconscious, or a cerebral mythology articulated onto a neurophysiological model: it is a place detached from consciousness, peopled with images and passions, shot through with discordances. In fact, the Freudian unconscious is a psychical, dynamic, and affective unconscious, organized through a number of functions (the ego, the id, and the superego).

Beyond this definition, the great Freudian innovation consists in a break with the idea of man as perpetually alienated. In this sense, Freud marks his distance as much from the alienation theory of Pinel as from the heirs of Mesmer. For while the Freudian subject can no longer be assimilated to the senseless animal so much feared by Couthon, nor is he that stranger to himself or herself defined by Pinel, whose soul must be tended through a "moral" treatment.

The Freudian subject is a free subject, endowed with reason, but a reason that vacillates inside itself. It is from her speech and actions, and not from her alienated consciousness, that the future possibility of her own cure will be able to emerge. This subject is not the automaton of the psychologists, nor the cerebrospinal individual of the physiologists, nor the somnambulist of the hypnotists, nor the ethical animal of the theorists of race and heredity. He or she is a speaking being, capable of analyzing the meaning of dreams rather than regarding them as the trace of a genetic memory.[25] Of course, the subject is limited by physical, chemical, or biological determinations but also by an unconscious conceived in terms of universality and singularity.

Freud was able to grant the unconscious a capacity for remembering and repression at the very moment when neurophysiology was throwing away the bases of a materialism of the body, making concrete the death of representations of the soul centered around the figure of god. Borne along by this kind of idea of the unconscious, psychoanalysis in the twentieth century was able to become the emblem of all the contemporary forms of exploration of subjectivity. Whence its impact on the other sciences, whence its permanent dialogue with religion and philosophy.

It is because Freud put subjectivity at the heart of his structure that he came to conceptualize an (unconscious) determination obliging the subject no longer to regard himself as master of the world but as a consciousness of self external to the spiral of mechanical causalities. In this sense, Freudian theory is certainly the heir of romanticism and a philosophy of critical liberty stemming from Kant and the Enlightenment philosophers. For it is the only one—and in this it also differs from all those that come from (unconscious, cerebral) physiology, from (unconscious, hereditary) biology, and from psychology (of the mind acting automatically)—to install the primacy of a subject inhabited by the consciousness of his own unconscious, or again by the consciousness of his own dispossession. In other words, the Freudian subject is possible only because it can think the existence of its unconscious: its particular unconscious. In the same way, the subject is only free because it agrees to take up the challenge of this constraining liberty and reconstructs its meaning.

Thus psychoanalysis is the only late-nineteenth-century psychological doctrine to have made a link between a philosophy of liberty and a theory of the psyche. It is in some sense an advance of civilization against barbarity. And this is why it was so successful for a century in countries marked by Western culture: in Europe, in the United States, in Latin America. Notwithstanding the attacks made on it, and notwithstanding the rigidity of its institutions, in these circumstances it ought once again today to be able to bring a humanist response to the gentle and death-dealing savagery of a depressive society tending to reduce human beings to machines without thought or feeling.

CHAPTER 6

The "Equinox Letter"

The Freudian unconscious rests on a paradox: the subject is free but has lost the mastery of his or her interiority, is no longer "master in his own house," in the well-known formula.[1] Freud disengages the subject from the different kinds of alienation to which it is tied by the other conceptions of psychology. In the same way, he constructs a theory of sexuality very different from all those that were advanced by scientists at the end of the nineteenth century.[2]

This novelty can be discovered through a reading of the famous "equinox letter," written on September 21, 1897, in which Freud explains the reasons why he is giving up the so-called seduction theory: "I no longer believe in my *neurotica*. . . . Now I can once again remain quiet and modest, go on worrying and saving. . . . 'Rebecca, take off your gown, you are no longer a bride.'"[3]

The word *seduction* refers first of all to the idea of a sexual scene where a subject, generally adult, uses his or her real or imaginary power to abuse another subject reduced to a position of passivity: a child or woman, mostly. The word is thus charged with the weight of an act based on the moral and physical violence exercised over another: executioner and victim, master and slave, dominant and dominated.

And when, from 1895 to 1897, Freud elaborates the famous theory that the origin of neurosis is in real sexual abuse, he does indeed start off from the the hypothesis of a traumatic alienation through having been forced. The theory depends as much on a social reality as on clinical evidence. In families, sometimes even in the street, children are often victims of offensive behavior on the part of adults. The memory of such brutalities is so unpleasant that everyone prefers to forget them, not to see them, or to repress them.

Through listening to turn-of-the-century hysterical women confiding stories like this to him, Freud is satisfied with their accounts and constructs his first hypothesis: that of repression and the sexual causality of hysteria. He thinks it is because they really have been seduced that hysterical women suffer from neurotic troubles. And so he starts having doubts about fathers in general, Jacob Freud in particular, but also himself: hadn't he experienced culpable desires in relation to his daughter Matilda?

It is through his contact with Wilhelm Fliess that Freud gradually abandons his seduction theory. He knows that not all fathers are rapists, but at the same time he allows that hysterics are not lying when they say they are victims of seduction attempts. How can these two contradictory truths be explained? Freud sets about it by taking a distance from the obvious. He perceives two things: first, that often the women invent the attacks in question, without lying or simulation, and, second, that when the event did indeed take place, it still does not explain the hatching of the neurosis. Freud therefore substitutes the theory of fantasy for that of seduction and by the same token resolves the enigma of sexual causes: they are fantasmatic, even when there is a real trauma, since the reality of fantasy is of a different nature from material reality.[4]

The abandonment of the notion of trauma as the sole type of cause goes together with the adoption of a psychical unconscious. In fact, the Freudian theory of sexuality assumes the prior existence of instinctual and fantasmatic sexual activity. It is based on the idea that the subject is both free of his or her sexuality and constrained by it. And above all it rejects the illusory project of getting rid of it, as if it were a question of a wrongdoing or the effect of a trauma.

Armed with these theories, Freud would always show himself to be fierce toward those, like Carl Gustav Jung, who abandoned the sexual theory for the "black tide of mud . . . of occultism":[5] "I am not expecting an immediate successor," he wrote to Ernest Jones, "but a perpetual battle. Anyone who promises humanity that he will liberate it from the trials of sex will be welcomed as a hero, he will be allowed to speak—whatever nonsense he spouts."[6]

In thus making sexuality and the unconscious the foundation of the subjective experience of freedom, Freud breaks with the religion of admission and confession as much as with the scientistic ideal of sexology: this new approach is neither a witch-hunt, nor a classification from on high, nor fascination with the kind of cheap eroticism characteristic of scientism or religious puritanism. For him, the point is not to judge sex or make it transparent or spectacular but to let it be expressed in the most normal and honest way. For nothing is further from the Freudian conception than the idea that sexuality is naturally unhealthy. Thus Freud is the inventor of a science of subjectivity that goes together with Western societies establishing notions of private life and legal subjects.

In the matter of sexuality, then, the Freudian scandal consists in reversing the order of normativity and in taking humanity's negativity for its positive nature. "The scandal," writes Michel Foucault, "is not in the fact that love should be naturally or originally sexual, which had been said before Freud, but in that through psychoanalysis, love, social relations, and the forms of belonging between people, appear as the negative element of sexuality inasmuch as sexuality is humanity's natural positivity."[7]

Freud's abandonment of the seduction theory also reminds us that the Viennese thinker's work was contemporary with the passing of the set of laws that cumulatively played a major part in the weakening of the power of the fathers in Western society: laws reducing paternal rights, laws on bad forms of treatment, on corporal punishment, and so forth.[8] In other words, Freud could only invent his theory in a world marked by the dislocation of traditional modes of familial organization. For as long as the father was vested with the law of an unlimited capacity enabling him to exercise a tyrannical power over the bodies of women and children, by repressing adultery on one side and masturbation on the other, no theorization of sexuality in terms of fantasy, memories, or conflict was possible.[9] This is why, everywhere in the world, psychoanalysis was to become an urban phenomenon affecting subjects sunk in anonymity, solitary or detached from their traditional attachments, and folded in on a restricted family nucleus.[10]

For the theory of seduction, we can outline three tendencies among Freudians and anti-Freudians.

The first, that of Freudian orthodoxy, is not interested in real seductions but overvalues fantasy. It leads to never being concerned during analysis with the real abuse suffered by the patient in his or her childhood or present life.

The second, represented at one extreme by the supporters of libertarian sexology and at the other by the puritans, tends to deny the existence of fantasy and take every form of psychical disturbance back to an actually lived trauma. For the libertarians, the actual practice of sex is an imperative: it is necessary for psychical health to flourish. As a result, abuse is a pedagogy of pleasure. For the puritans, on the contrary, all sexuality is reduced to an act of abuse.

As for the third tendency, the only one to conform to psychoanalytic thought and to straightforward good sense, it consists of accepting the existence of both fantasy and trauma linked to sexual abuse. Clinically, a psychoanalyst thus has to be capable of telling the difference between the two orders of reality, often interlocked, and of understanding that psychical violence or emotional torture can be experienced as being as terrible as sexual abuse.[11] In other words, denying fantasy risks provoking in a subject an injury as mutilating as the denial of a real act of abuse.[12]

To go further: If one remains dependent on the seduction theory, one risks thinking that a trauma is in itself responsible for a definitive destruction of the one who has undergone it. In this sense, the cult of victimhood is the equivalent of biological determinism, letting it be understood that children who have been maltreated by the people around them or assaulted in extreme circumstances (war, terrorism, etc.) are bound to become delinquents or complain perpetually of an injury that cannot be healed. It was against this tenacious prejudice that Freud protested when he gave up his theory. Nothing is ever played out in advance: the misfortune is not inscribed in the genes or the neurones. All subjects have a history of their own that makes them react differently from someone else in identical situations. Consequently, a real trauma is not in itself more murderous than serious psychical suffering.

Psychoanalysis linked a nongenital theory of sexuality to a noncerebral conception of the unconscious and made a distinction between trauma and fantasy so as to conceptualize them in their difference; that is why it was considered a form of pansexualism throughout the first half of the twentieth century. Its opponents feared its possible impact on the social body and accused it of introducing moral disorder into the family.

In Latin countries, psychoanalysis was treated as a barbaric science born of Teutonic decadence, and in Nordic countries it was regarded as the sign of a Latin degeneration; but in puritan countries, and particularly in Canada and the United States, it was designated as a Satanic doctrine. To put this another way, the antisexual hatred aroused by psychoanalysis was both a symptom of its growing success and a sign of the sexual and psychical emancipation of which it was the promise. To this accusation of pansexualism, some added that of pansymbolism: they accused Freud of having restored a spiritualist conception of the unconscious based on an art of divination—the decoding of symbols and dreams—a long way from scientific rationality.[13]

CHAPTER 7

Freud Is Dead in America

In the years following World War II, at a time when psychoanalysis was enjoying great success in the United States and a revival in France and developing fast in Latin America, it went on being attacked. The pansexualism argument fell into disuse in parallel with transformations to the family and the emancipation of women. But with the success of psychotropic drugs and the medical advances achieved, it was becoming possible to challenge the status of the Freudian unconscious.

As a result, a new cerebral mythology established itself with the aim of demonstrating that psychoanalysis was not a science but a method of literary introspection or a variant of the ancient key to dreams. This mythology took the name cognitive unconscious.[1] For its supporters, it was indeed about reviving the idea of a possible fit between the brain and thought, based on an analogy between brain functioning and the computer.

Cognitive science appeared in the United States around 1950. The initial task it set itself was to describe the dispositions and capacities of the human mind (cognition), such as language, perception, reasoning, motor coordination, and planning. Resting on a conception of the mind according to which the mental and the neural are two sides of a single phenomenon, this "science" also used a number of fast-developing disciplines: neurobiology, or the study of chemical mediators explaining human behavior down to the most basic element of the human organism, namely the gene; neurophysiology, which was interested in the functional significance of the properties of the brain; artificial intelligence, which studied reasoning by taking the computer as the model of brain functioning; and neuropsychology, or the description of pathological phenomena linked to the functioning of cognition. The aim of all these disciplines was, and still is, to give a universal account of the functioning of human mental activity starting from a characterization of the nervous system as a physico-chemical system.[2]

The primary objective of this cognitive psychology was to contest first behaviorism, but above all psychoanalysis, considered as a real plague.[3] Howard Gardner writes:

> There was also the intoxication of psychoanalysis. While many scholars were intrigued by Freud's intuitions, they felt that no scientific discipline could be constructed on the basis of clinical interviews and retrospectively constructed personal histories; moreover they deeply resented the pretense of a field that did not leave itself susceptible to disconfirmation. Between the "hard line" credo of the Establishment behaviorists and the unbridled conjecturing of the Freudians, it was difficult to focus in a scientifically respectable way on the territory of human thought processes.[4]

In fact, there is an important difference between cognitive psychology—which wants to be scientific, claiming that not only the production of thought, but also conscious and unconscious psychical organization, are dependent on the brain—and the scientific disciplines (or neurosciences) that it is based on. The idea that what the human mind does can be achieved in the same way by a machine (the computer) comes from Alan Turing, the brilliant inventor of the machine that bears his name.[5] Yet, as we have seen, a good many neurobiologists refuse this aberrant hypothesis, which is nonetheless the very essence of the new cerebral mythology of the cognitivists. "One day," writes Gerald Edelman, "the most visible practitioners of cognitive psychology and the most arrogant empirical neurobiologists will finally understand that they have unwittingly been the victims of an intellectual con-trick."[6]

Here are a few examples, out of hundreds, of so-called scientific analyses put forward by the supporters of cognitivism.

In a 1996 lecture that partly restates the thesis of his book,[7] the American anthropologist Lawrence Hirschfeld tries to resolve a supposed enigma: through what cognitive processes do American children of "white" race nowadays internalize what is known as "the one-drop-of-blood rule" when the notion of race has been banished since 1950 from all the natural sciences, human sciences, and social sciences?[8] Universally shared, this rule correlates the imaginary notion of race with the manifestation of a pure biological difference: skin color. It thus perpetuates the belief according to which race is a stigma inscribed on the body in the form of a cutaneous variation. As a result, "black blood" present in a white child born of a mixed marriage would automatically make him or her the bearer of the invisible trace of a blackness that he could then transmit to his offspring by engendering children of "black" race.

Hirschfeld distinguishes between two interpretations of the famous rule. The first is "categorial" and depends on a racial and therefore racist conception of humanity; the second is "biological" and relies on the scientific idea that the human species is not made up of races but of human groups that are physically different from one another (blacks, whites, Asiatics, etc.).

Armed with this interpretation and a battery of tests, Hirschfeld then divides his interlocutors (white and American) into three groups: seven-year-old children, eleven-year-old children, and adults. He gives each group two images, one showing "uniracial" couples and the other "interracial" couples, consisting of either a black man and a white woman or a a white man and a black woman. When asked about the offspring of these couples, all the interlocutors, whatever their age, reply that the children born of the uniracial couples will necessarily belong to the same race as their parents and have the same physical characteristics as each of them.

In contrast, the questionnaire on the interracial couples produces divergent responses. The majority of the seven-year-olds are unable to give an opinion about physical resemblances, though they do declare that the child of a mixed couple will necessarily belong to the same race as its mother. But the eleven-year-olds expect this same child to bear a physical resemblance to its black parent (father or mother), without however belonging to any particular race. As for the adults, they think that any child born to an interracial couple will be racially black, even if it resembles its white parent.

Hirschfeld's conclusion from this experiment is that the adoption of the "categorial" (racist) version of the rule of the drop of blood depends on a distinctive process that occurs spontaneously as the child grows up and becomes an adult. In other words, instead of asking why seven-year-old children always privilege maternal capacity above physical appearance and why, in contrast, eleven-year-olds privilege a balance between the two poles (maternal and paternal) above membership of a race and instead, finally, of trying to understand why white American adults assimilate a physical difference to a race, Hirschfeld is content to announce, with the aid of a battery of tests that prove nothing, that the perception of race must be a natural element of human cognition. As a result, the racist attitude must be an immovable and universal structure on which individuals' political and cultural choices are dependent.

It will then come as no surprise that Fannie Hurst's famous novel *Imitation of Life*, which inspired this experiment, should be more relevant than Hirschfeld's convoluted jargon to interpret the profound significance of the great American myth of the drop of blood.[9] A long way from all the would-be experimentation on whether racial feeling is innate or acquired, the work retraces the tragic existence of a white woman unconsciously suffering from the anguish of biological pollution who chooses sterilization as a solution to her identity fantasy rather than having to confront the risk of transmitting the invisible stigmata of the hated race to her offspring.

As to the question of knowing why a belief persists after it has been invalidated by science, I won't dwell on that now.

If Lawrence Hirschfeld applies cognitive science to the domain of anthropology, Howard Gardner, the American assailant of psychoanalysis, has recourse to the same doctrine for his invention of a would-be "science of exceptionality." In one of his studies, published in 1997, he thinks he can explain the genesis of genius in four great "personalities"—Mozart, Freud, Gandhi, and Virginia Woolf—by constructing a typology of characteristics and forms of behavior that you would think had come straight out of a mixture of astrology and folkloric psychology. So we have Mozart as the prototype of the Master because, thanks to his mental faculties, he knew how to acquire "perfect mastery of the genres of his time"; Freud as the "Model Builder" (or MB), because, through his parents' love, he had the benefit of "comfortable working conditions"; and Gandhi as the very type of the Charismatic because he knew how to influence those who resisted pacifism and convert them to his ideas. Finally, we have Virginia Woolf as the best incarnation of the Introspective, because, having suffered abuse in her childhood, she was able to turn her gaze inside herself, to understand the human race.[10]

With figures to support him and a proliferation of charts, graphics, and measurements of every kind, Gardner thus constructs, in all seriousness, his psychology of typical profiles on the basis of which he thinks he can explain exceptional destinies by contrasting them with ordinary fates. In other words, the "science" we are dealing with here bears no relation to the scientific approach.

Christopher Frith, an English researcher and professor of neuropsychology, proposes to explain the genesis of schizophrenia by showing it to be "an alteration of the processes implicated in the initiation of action": poverty of action, in some way linked to a failure in the central (cerebral) control of communication (central monitoring system).[11] This form of madness has been known since time immemorial but was described in 1911 by Bleuler. It is characterized by splitting—incoherence of thought, affectivity, and action—to which may be added delirious activity and withdrawal into the self. All these symptoms are united in delusions of control that lead the patient to think he or she is dominated in his thoughts and actions by diabolical forces outside him.

But for Frith, schizophrenia is only a failure of "mentalization" brought on by physico-chemical processes themselves malfunctioning and not connected to a delirious organization, though they do indicate the psychical reality.

Supporters of all these theses, flourishing in the laboratories of contemporary scientific research, seem to be unaware of the famous story of the madman who leaves the asylum dragging behind him a funnel attached to a string. When the well-meaning guard asks him how his dog is, he replies: "But it isn't a dog, it's a funnel!" A few yards further on, once he has passed the entrance to the hospital, he turns round and calls to the object: "Hey, Mirza, we fooled him all right, didn't we?"

What all these theories have in common is to support a reactionary and nihilistic vision of humanity. No point in fighting racism, because what you are dealing with is an innate disposition inscribed in the neurones. No point in researching the meaning of the distinctive history of one particular person—genius, talented, or ordinary—if that history is a matter of necessity. No point, finally, in getting preoccupied with the meaning of what is said by the mentally ill, if the person afflicted by madness is only cognitively disabled; to treat him, surely all we need do is classify his symptoms in the *DSM* category most appropriate to his behavior and then treat him with the corresponding antipsychotic drugs? The best one can do is to try, with the help of diverse injunctions, to persuade him to stop his false reasoning.

There is no direct link between the development of the cognitive sciences and the *DSM*'s dismantling of the four great models of dynamic psychiatry, but it was certainly in the name of the same assumptions that the great cleaning-up operation was effected, for both of these and at the same time, with the aim of eradicating the whole group of theories of subjectivity from academic and medical thought. And among these theories, the one most targeted was obviously psychoanalysis, inasmuch as the Freudian conception of the unconscious was fundamentally incompatible with the new mythology of the brain.

In this context, there is an important difference between the situation of psychoanalysis in the United States and in France.

While it was possible to save psychoanalysis from Nazism through the large-scale emigration of European Freudians to the North American continent between 1930 and 1940, the price was a radical transformation of its ideals, its practice, and its theory. From the beginning of the century, it was welcomed as a theology of individual fulfillment: a healthy soul in a healthy body. The extremely pragmatic American therapists enthusiastically seized hold of Freudian ideas. But they straightaway sought to measure sexual energy, to prove the efficacy of analyses by producing endless statistics and conducting surveys to find out whether the concepts could be applied empirically to the concrete problems of individuals.

In these circumstances, and with all tendencies mixed up, transatlantic psychoanalysis became the instrument of an adaptation of humanity to a utopia of happiness. It won recognition less for its system of thought or for the philosophical questionings it brought with it than for its capacity to offer an immediate solution to the sexual morality of a liberal and puritan society. Through psychoanalysis, the "guilty" person was no longer condemned to the hell of his passions but capable of freeing himself from them; thanks to it, he would no longer be constrained by a diabolical sexuality, he could detach himself from it. Yet, as I have already stressed, nothing is more foreign to Freudian thought than this healthy ideal that assumes that sexuality is unwholesome and that the normal individual must make a confession about it in order to erase the trace of an original sin from his mind.

Fritz Wittels, a Viennese disciple of Freud's who had become an American citizen, wrote an extremely lucid chapter on this subject in his *Memoirs*:

> The soil in which psychoanalysis grew and expanded has been destroyed—for a century. Its future depends entirely on America, which means that either there will be no psychoanalysis in the future, or it will have to thrive in America. . . . May the expression of a few misgivings regarding this future therefore be permitted.
>
> America's magnificent scientific spirit is as yet devoted to dimensions, to measuring and weighing, to figures and statistics. . . . [Americans] can understand the highest buildings as such, the longest aqueducts, the deepest chasms. . . . They wish to have the costliest paintings in the biggest museums or in the mansions of the richest men. They are less qualified for a scientific approach to the irrational world of the soul, which they either reject as not scientific, or accept in the form of pseudoscientific, typically American doctrines like Christian Science, Buchmanism[12] or, further West, as evangelical doctrine from the lips of white-robed priestesses.[13]

After having been used for about thirty years as cement for the elaboration of psychiatric nosology, psychoanalysis was finally rejected: didn't psychotropic drugs and the other explanatory models of the mind, based on *DSM IV* or on new mythologies of the brain, offer faster therapeutic solutions to those well-known "disorders" that imprisoned the subject in a behavioral symptomatology? In this way, as the historian Nathan Hale brings out very well, the advocates of American anti-Freudianism of the 1970s and 1980s went back to using against psychoanalysis the same methods that Freudian enthusiasts had employed at the start of the century.[14] They, too, proposed evaluations, proofs, efficiency surveys: in short, a whole experimentalist arsenal unsuitable for taking account of the reality of psychoanalytic theory and practice.

Freud was aware of these drifts and expressed his hostility many times in the form of a fairly basic anti-Americanism. In one letter to Wittels, he insisted: "These primitives have little interest in science which is not directly convertible into practice. The worst of the American way is their so-called broadmindedness through which they even feel themselves to be superior to us narrowminded Europeans." And in another: "Sure, the American and psychoanalysis are often so ill-adapted for one another that one is reminded of Grabbe's parable, 'as though a raven were to put on a white shirt.'"[15]

The most representative attitude in today's scientistic crusade is that of Adolf Grünbaum. A well-known physicist, a philosopher, and then a professor of psychiatry, he became a specialist in anti-Freudianism around 1970. In his 1984 book *The Foundations of Psychoanalysis*, which caused a huge stir in the United States, he picked up again the classical argument of advocates of the brain mythology, reproaching Freud for having abandoned his *Project* and given up on making psychoanalysis a natural science.[16] To bolster his argument, Grünbaum attacked the theses of three philosophers who, so he said, had completely misunderstood the Freudian approach: Karl Popper, Paul Ricoeur, and Jürgen Habermas.[17] He objected to Popper's claim that psychoanalysis was "irrefutable" in relation to science since it could never be subjected to tests of refutability in the same way as the other natural sciences. He criticized what he saw as Ricoeur's mistaken attitude toward Freud: for Ricoeur, Freud had wanted to make psychoanalysis into a science but had not understood that it would always remain a "hermeneutics of the depths" associated with a method of reflection about oneself. Last, Grünbaum accused Habermas of having transformed psychoanalysis into a hermeneutics cut off from any experimental anchoring.

In short, Grünbaum was extremely angry with a philosophical discourse (Popper, Ricoeur, Habermas) that had been concerned either to criticize the ambivalences of Freudian scientism or to valorize a model that excluded the subject from the domain of science. As I have already stressed, Freud was always tempted, *even though he gave this up* from 1896, to make psychoanalysis a natural science, in accordance with which the unconscious would be purely a product of brain functioning. The fact that he abandoned this project, even as he continued to dream about it, obviously does not mean that he refused to make psychoanalysis a scientific discipline. And indeed it is precisely for this reason that he adopted a critical attitude toward the mythologies of the brain that was much more scientific than that of the scientists.[18]

Against this philosophical discourse, Grünbaum thus claimed that the Freudian dream had to be taken literally.

But the substance of what he was saying was that since Freud had had the nerve to abandon true science before even constructing his system of thought, then the whole lot of his concepts should be left behind on the grounds of non-scientificity. There followed a set-piece demolition of all the hypotheses of psychoanalysis: its clinical method is a fraud, reproducing a placebo effect; its metaphysical construction betrays a vast program of interpretive totalitarianism based on attributing an arbitrary meaning to actions or thoughts; last, the quarrels among its different branches are just the expression of denominational fanaticisms with no intellectual validity. And Grünbaum was as angry with Freud as with his successors (Winnicott and Kohut), accused, like their master, of being pseudoscholars.

In fact, the physicist was making tendentious use of the surveys evaluating psychoanalysis that had been conducted in the United States from 1952. These surveys, as we have seen,[19] do not make it possible to decide the question of whether psychoanalysis is superior to the other forms of psychotherapy. But they do offer proof that psychical forms of treatment, taking all tendencies together, are extremely effective (80 percent "successful"). As a result, they constitute the proof that Grünbaum's fanatical anti-Freudianism is in no way scientific.

On the question of experimental validation, Grünbaum limited himself to demolishing one of Freud's great case histories: the Rat Man, whose real name was Ernst Lanzer.[20]

During the analysis, Freud had connected the fear of rats with a childhood memory recounted by Lanzer, who had been punished by his father for masturbating. Commenting on this passage, Grünbaum suspected Freud of taking what the patient said literally and believing in this childhood episode that perhaps had never existed. Then he objected to his establishing a relation of cause and effect between the fear of rats and obsessional neurosis. In short, he accused him of inventing a system of interpretation that bore no relation to reality.

It would of course be possible to oppose Grünbaum with another argument drawn from another Freudian analysis, that of the Wolf Man, whose real name was Sergueï Constantinovitch Pankejeff.

During this analysis, Freud had reconstructed a primal scene on the basis of his patient's dream. At the age of eighteen months, Sergueï had seen his parents, on their knees on the white bed sheets, indulging in intercourse *a tergo* three times over. Questioned about this many years later, Pankejeff declared that presumably this scene had never taken place, since in Russia children do not sleep in their parents' bedroom. But he added straight away that the primal scene reconstructed by Freud had taken on an immense truth-value for him. Finally, he stressed that psychoanalysis had been the only and the first treatment, after many spells of hospitalization, to relieve him from his distress and give a meaning to his existence.[21]

If this example shows that Freud can on occasion construct an imaginary scene so as to enable the patient to accede to his own history, another example attests that he did once imagine a scene that had really happened.

Around 1925, from the start of her analysis, Marie Bonaparte recounts to Freud a dream in which she sees herself, in her cradle, in the presence of scenes of intercourse. By way of interpretation, Freud declares in a peremptory tone that she not only heard these scenes, like most children who sleep in

their parents' bedroom, but that she saw them in broad daylight. Being a very different kind of character from Sergueï
Pankejeff, Marie Bonaparte rejects this statement, protesting
that she never had a mother. Freud stands his ground, coun-
tering this with the presence of the nurse. Anxious for experimental proofs, the princess then decides to interrogate
her father's half-brother, who had looked after the horses at
the house they had lived in during her childhood. By speaking about the elevated scientific scope of psychoanalysis in
front of him, she gets him to admit his long-ago liaison with
the nurse. And the old man tells how once upon a time he
had made love in broad daylight in front of Marie's cradle.
So she had indeed witnessed scenes of fellatio, intercourse,
and cunnilingus.[22]

These clinical histories are a good indication of the disjunction Freud brings about between knowledge and truth.
Like Socrates, he actualizes the idea that it is in dialogue that
the subject discovers what was repressed: the primal scene,
inasmuch as it is at the origin of his existence and of the difference of the sexes. So it hardly matters whether or not this
scene was invented since it articulates the truth of an original
structure that sets each person face to face with his destiny
and with the tragedy of his desire. Let us go further: this
scene draws its signifying force from being constructed. Now
it is precisely this disjunction, verifiable as it is in the accounts
of analyses and in patients' testimonies, that is inadmissible
for the supporters of scientism, who always make the intel-
lect coincide with the thing and knowledge with the truth.
For the same reasons, moreover, they conceive of human behavior as a pattern and the brain as a producer of cogito. In
doing this, they are committing a scientific error. They are in

fact taking experimentation to be the only proof of a subjective truth, without ever perceiving the difference between the natural sciences and the human sciences.

It is obvious that biologists or physicists don't have to get the gene, the atom, or the molecule to intervene in their work. Yet supporters of scientist and the mythologies of the brain act as if brain physiology could be interrogated like a subject capable of speaking the truth of an existential lived experience.

To understand the impasse that an approach like this leads to, it is sufficient to quote the testimony of Corinne Hamon, a French psychiatrist and psychoanalyst: "A patient came to see me in a state of depression that had been going on for a very long time. A whole load of GPs had treated her. I had an interview with her, and I gave her antidepressants. It takes five or six days for this medication to have an effect. But the very next day, her husband phoned me to say she was feeling much better. She had been listened to in a way she never had been before. She was able to leave behind something of her depression and ask herself questions about herself that she never had."[23]

The end point of Grünbaum's fundamentalism was the liquidation of every form of argumentation not based on the statement of a fact. And this is why at the end of his book the author devoted himself to dubious speculation about the question of seduction. To grasp its significance, it is essential to understand the issues in the Freudian problematic of sexuality.

We have seen that the condition of emergence of a Freudian theory of subjective liberty rested as much on abandoning various mythologies of the brain elaborated at the end of

the nineteenth century as on giving up an explanation of psychical causality purely in terms of trauma. Whence the event
of 1897 and the famous "equinox letter": Freud's abandonment of the theory of seduction. Now, at the moment when,
in the United States, the scientistic slide of the 1980s was
leading to the breakdown of the Freudian model of the unconscious, another form of madness, this one puritanical,
was attacking another major conception of the Freudian system: the theory of fantasy.

In 1980 Kurt Eissler, curator of the Sigmund Freud Archives
(SFA), and Anna Freud decided to entrust the complete publication of Freud's letters to Fliess to an American academic
who had been duly trained in the inner circle of the International Psychoanalytic Association (IPA). Jeffrey Moussaieff
Masson got to know the archives by interpreting them in a
crude way, with the idea that they were hiding a hidden
truth, a shameful secret. This was how he came to assert,
without any kind of proof, that Freud had given up the seduction theory out of cowardice. Not daring to reveal to the
world the atrocities committed by all adults on all children,
Freud invented the notion of fantasy to mask the traumatic
reality of sexual abuse at the origin of neuroses. So he was
quite simply a forger.

   In 1984 Masson published a book on this subject, *The
Assault on Truth*, which was one of the biggest American
psychoanalytic best-sellers of the second half of the century.[24] Against the orthodoxies of the theory of fantasy, the
work served to reinforce the theses of revisionist historiography.[25] The point was to show that the Freudian lie had
perverted the United States by allying itself with a power

based on oppression: colonization of women by men, of children by adults, and of natural vivacity by concepts, and so on.

Although it had been strongly criticized by the majority of feminist movements, the thesis of traumatic seduction again appeared as the only solution to the enigma of a sexuality that had once more become brutal and detestable. Like Masson, the famous lawyer Catherine MacKinnon took up the idea of the Freudian lie. She was a specialist in sexual harassment trials, while seeking to establish the principle that all women, in childhood or in their adult lives, had been victims of acts of abuse on the part of men. She even proposed to utilize various procedures—inquisitorial investigations, persuasion, hypnosis, psychopharmacology, and others—in order to rediscover the traces of a repressed seduction in subjects' unconscious minds. Whence the claim that sexuality is in itself and always an assault on women's bodies. In 1992 Judith Herman published a book revising the history of hysteria in line with a revalorization of trauma. The first stage, according to the author, was when hysteria emerged in the discourse of Charcot as an echo of French republicanism. It was then emancipated in 1920 with the collapse of the cult of war and the deployment of pacifism, before finally, in the context of the feminist movement, revealing itself as nothing but traumatic sexual violence.[26]

The abandonment of the theory of fantasy for a return to the seduction theory went together with a revalorization of an unconscious thought of in terms of dissociation and mental automatism. As a result, there was a considerable increase in multiple personality syndrome in the United States, as *DSM III* and *DSM IV* adopted a terminology from which Freud and Bleuler's nosology had disappeared.

Defined as a disturbance of identity, the phenomenon of multiple personality developed in the nineteenth century before disappearing around 1910, at the moment when, under the influence of the second type of dynamic psychiatry and the Freudian conception of neurosis, women, who formed the majority of the sufferers, were regarded as full subjects and no longer as strange, sexually abused, and hampered by a dislocated consciousness. Henri F. Ellenberger gives a remarkable description of the syndrome, which gave rise to numerous literary narratives.[27] Clinically, it manifested itself in the coexistence in a subject of one or a number of personalities separated from each other, each of them able to take control in its turn. In 1972 the notion seemed like a curiosity from another age. Only a dozen or so cases had been recorded since 1920. Yet the number of patients having this syndrome since 1986 is estimated at six thousand. In 1992 it was thought that one in twenty people were suffering from the disturbance, to the point that there were clinics in all North American cities that specialized in the treatment of the new epidemic.[28]

This phenomenal increase certainly proves the regression in nosology brought about by the various revisions of the *DSM*. It is because they no longer came under a meaningful classification that women patients with hysterical disturbances or psychoses then received a diagnosis of multiple personality. The syndrome does indeed reflect a model of society in which the woman is assimilated to a sexually abused victim suffering from despair about her identity.

In the wake of the Masson affair, the U.S. revisionist current set about dismantling Freudian doctrine and Freud himself, once again become a diabolical scientist guilty of indulging in abusive relationships within his own family. As early as 1981 Peter Swales was claiming—without a shred of proof, of course—that Freud had had a sexual relationship with his sister-in-law Minna Bernays, and even that he had got her pregnant and forced her to have an abortion.

Revisionist historiography, which made its appearance around 1978, had initially been very creative. Researchers taking their lead from it, thinking of themselves as the heirs of the great historian Henri F. Ellenberger, had produced some remarkable work: this was particularly true of Frank Sulloway, author of a monumental work on the biological origins of Freudian thought.[29] These historians justifiably challenged the canons of official history, inherited from Ernest Jones and above all from Kurt Eissler, after World War II the principal organizer of the SFA deposited in the Library of Congress in Washington, D.C. But after a few years of heated fighting against Freudian orthodoxy, the revisionist current became so anti-Freudian that it gave up scholarly studies to launch itself fanatically into the war of ideas.[30]

In the 1990s context, the hypotheses of some revisionists were an absolute godsend for the supporters of scientism, who, however, did not share them. What they did was to reinforce the idea that a trauma, meaning a trace that was visible and thus assumed to be inscribed in the memory, could explain subjective disorders. Whence the potential linkup between a clinical practice seeking to explore the human brain to find the origin of a pathology and a coercive psychology sometimes based on hypnosis, sometimes on psychopharmacology, and making it possible to replace psychoanalysis with a technology of confession or a behaviorist type of symptomatological evaluation.

Two case histories, from millions of others, testify to the scale of the manic quest for sexual abuse and multiple personality at the moment when, with the fall of communism and the absence of any counterpower, U.S. society seemed to have delivered itself body and soul to the triple grasp of scientism, liberalism, and the demonization of sex.

The first is that of a nineteen-year-old student who had a conflicted relationship with her father and whose existence became agonizing at the end of 1989. Showing symptoms of depression and bulimia, including a hatred of bananas, *fromage frais*, and mayonnaise, she decided, with her parents' agreement, to undertake a treatment in a medical center catering to the well-off. She was taken in hand by a psychologist responsible for relations with the family and a psychiatrist and was immediately put in the category of "sexually abused women." This diagnosis was put forward by the psychiatrist on the basis of a hypothesis that in 80 percent of cases bulimia is a symptom of sexual abuse that took place in childhood or adolescence.

Yet this hypothesis is entirely wrong. All the studies on bulimia demonstrate that, as one symptom among others, its origin, depending on its seriousness, may be psychical, hormonal, or genetic. And it appears in many types of situations—in patients who are depressive, hysterical, perverse, hypochondriac, schizophrenic, and so on—and in no case implies, as such, the existence of sexual abuse.[31]

After the treatment had gone on for some time, the young woman brought up vague memories of being touched by her father, without being more specific. Obsessed with the idea of detecting a tangible proof of sexual abuse, the psychiatrist then decided to administer a truth drug (sodium amytal) to his patient, in order to get the repressed memories to emerge. Under the effect of the drug, the young woman recounted extravagant scenes: in her childhood, her father used to rape her and force her to perform fellatio on him and on the family dog. Carried away by their interpretive delirium, the two therapists then declared that these recovered memories explained the patient's aversion to *fromage frais*, bananas, and mayonnaise. The refusal of these three delicacies was clearly, they said, the manifest symptom of sexual abuse.

Urged by her therapists, the young woman told the "truth" to her mother. The mother got a divorce and custody of the children, whereas the father, overcome by these "revelations" and by the gossip that was calling him a pedophile, lost his job. The case ended up in the courts. The father lodged a complaint against the therapists, and his lawyers, paid a fortune, called on experts specializing in the hunt for manipulators of false memory known to have destroyed the lives of well over ten thousand American families. Between reports and counterreports from experts, the jury was persuaded, by ten votes to two, that this man had never had sexual relations with his daughter. Supported by her mother, the daughter, however, reaffirmed what she had said. The court meanwhile sentenced the psychiatrist and the psychologist to a severe fine for "grave negligence" occurring "without harmful intent."[32]

"Without harmful intent": we see here how sorcerers' apprentices, with endless qualifications and haunted by the madness of experimentation and sexual abuse, thought they were authorized to enter by force and penetrate into another person's unconscious. The result of this disastrous case, in which the difference Freud established between trauma and fantasy was completely blurred, is that neither the patient nor her family will ever be able to know the truth of her history. And so she will remain the victim of a system itself based on a victimological delirium and the spread of scientistic ideology.

The second story, which goes back to the same period, is that of a woman who, with the help of the *DSM*, had been diagnosed with multiple personality disorder. When she was sexually attacked by a man and took the case to court, the lawyer for the prosecution maintained that she had twenty-one personalities and none of them had consented to having sex. The jury and the psychiatrists then had a discussion to ascertain whether this woman's different personalities would be capable of testifying under oath, and whether or not each of them had her own sexual adventures. In 1990 the man was found guilty because three of the victim's personalities had testified against him. But following a counterreport, a new trial took place. What had happened was that a number of psychiatrists had claimed that the lady had forty-six personalities rather than twenty-one. So it was necessary to find out whether these new personalities would also testify during the trial. . . .[33]

Cases like these have become frequent in North America. They show very well the kind of fanaticism that can result from the idea that any sexual act is in itself a sin, a rape, a trauma and any unconscious a dissociated state with no place for subjectivity.

In spite of these drifts, it should never be forgotten that it was this America that Freud so detested that also gave psychoanalysis its finest hours of glory after saving it from Nazism. And it was in the United States that the best scholarship on the history of Freudianism and Freud himself was published, as shown by the works of Peter Gay, Carl Schorske,

Nathan Hale, Ysef Hayim Yerushalmi, and plenty of others, too. No country has ever been so enthusiastic about the Viennese invention, and there have never been more supporters of psychical therapy. And doubtless this enthusiasm is not unrelated to the anti-Freudian rage that is manifesting itself at the dawn of the new century.

To close this chapter, I will return to Adolf Grünbaum, the principal U.S. representative of scientistically inspired anti-Freudianism. In his book, he ends up not deciding between the supporters of libertarian sexology, favorable to pedophiles, and the puritans, who reduce the sexual act to a form of abuse. He does this not to make clear the strange theoretical proximity of their respective attitudes, but to set against them the idea that only experimental testing, with calculations and samples, would make it possible to say whether or not subjects abused in their childhood are in a worse state as adults than others who have not lived through this drama.

Grünbaum never wonders about the nature of the malaise of abused subjects as opposed to those who have not been and who can, in some cases, present much more disturbing symptoms than those resulting from sexual cruelty. It is quite obvious that approaches of this type, where the object is to take stock of a psychical state rather than to understand its specific meaning, have no scientific value, since they do not take account of the reality of the state of the subject.

But there is a more serious problem than this: by adopting a so-called objective attitude, you condemn yourself to observing crimes (rape), offenses (pedophilia), transgressions (incest between adults), and straightforward neuroses all in the same way, and without making any distinctions between them. Scientistic objectivity is then just the screen behind which hides the thrill of abolishing any human relation to the Law and so to the Forbidden.

To satisfy this crazy rambling, will we one day have to shut up two groups of young children in laboratory cages, one accompanied by pedophiles and the other supervised by educators beyond suspicion? And then will we have to wait for a number of years to observe the differences and measure the gaps so as to conclude, after much hesitation, that traumatic effects either exist or are absent?

CHAPTER 8

A French Scientism

In France, scientistic hostility toward psychoanalysis never took on the appearance of such a furious conflict. For the first half of the century, attacks essentially polarized over Freudian "pansexualism," always assimilated to a "Teutonic" decadence. The enemies of the new doctrine deliberately treated it as "Kraut science" and judged it incapable of conveying the subtlety of the Latin or Cartesian genius. Faced with this situation, a number of pioneers tried to "Frenchify" psychoanalysis. This was particularly true of Edouard Pichon, the only one to give some coherence to this illusory project. As opposed to chauvinism, the surrealists—led by André Breton—proclaimed their attachment to a romantic conception of the unconscious.

At any rate, in France the resistance to psychoanalysis never took the exclusive form of scientism, and this tendency remained a minority one despite every effort on the part of representatives of psychology who missed no opportunity to denounce the nonexperimental nature of Freudian analysis. As to psychoanalytic doctrine, in France it was never taken as an ideology of happiness, but as the instrument criticizing all attempts to normalize subjectivity.

After World War II, the themes of pansexualism and Frenchness became obsolete. Debates between the propsychoanalytic and the antipsychoanalytic then took an ideological, political, or philosophical turn. Violently attacked by the Communist

Party between 1948 and 1956, psychoanalysis also became a target for the Catholic Church. And then, from the second half of the 1960s, the hostilities ceased. With support from Louis Althusser's thinking, the French communists revised their positions.[1] The Catholic Church meanwhile was forced into a compromise because of the spread of therapeutic practice among priests. Elsewhere, partly through the teaching of Jacques Lacan, the main arguments took place on the terrain of a psychiatry dominated by psychoanalytic clinical practice and in a context where philosophers and anthropologists, from Sartre to Merleau-Ponty, then from Lévi-Strauss to Foucault and Derrida, had been taking Freudian concepts as an object of reflection.[2]

It was thus possible for a new section of the human sciences to get started, whose principal concern was to elucidate the Freudian notion of the unconscious. For the existentialist philosophers, the interrogation focused on the compatibility between unconscious determination and subjective freedom, whereas for the structuralists the question was about knowing whether or not Freud's instinctual unconscious could be disengaged from biology to enter the frame of a general theory of symbolic systems.

During this period, the only French book comparable to Grünbaum's—and it was quite influential—was Pierre Debray-Ritzen's *La Scolastique freudienne* [Freudian scholasticism].[3] Debray-Ritzen was a child psychiatrist and hospital doctor; the position he adopted against psychoanalysis was as fanatical as that of his U.S. counterpart. He blamed Freud in the name of science for having abandoned the *Project* and the natural sciences to become the artisan of a new hermeneutics characterized as "scholastical." Treating hysteria as a "neuronal" illness and a "profound posturing" and claiming that schizophrenia was reducible to a genetic anomaly, he countered the Freudian unconscious with the culturalists' notion of pattern, and the theory of fantasy with that of trauma. Finally, he stressed that dreams have no meaning apart from the one invented by the therapist to con the patient.

Not content with treating Freud as a charlatan, Debray-Ritzen attacked Melanie Klein (described as "mad") and René Spitz. And to explain the affective failings of children abandoned in orphanages, he had no hesitation in appealing to genetic causes. Debray-Ritzen had links with the French Far Right, especially with the New Right, and enlivened his scientistic language with a "moral": in fact, he laid into divorce and abortion as well as Judeo-Christian religion, which he claimed was hostile to the fulfillment of the true materialist science. Whence the advocacy of a deranged atheism based on the cult of paganism.

If Debray-Ritzen's arguments were the same as those of the supporters of cerebral man, their political bases were different. And moreover, in later anti-Freudian developments—those of Jean-Pierre Changeux, Marcel Gauchet, or the French cognitivists—we never find such a radical tearing apart of Freud's oeuvre. Most of the time, the critiques are directed against the psychoanalytic conception of the unconscious. But in France it is as if Freud the man were in some sense beyond attack.

There is however one thing in common between the partisans of scientism and those of the reduction of the psyche to the neural, from Grünbaum to Debray-Ritzen to Changeux: an absolute rejection of religion. This atheism, it must obviously be pointed out, bears no resemblance to that of Freud or the heirs of the Enlightenment. Nor is it inspired by Renaissance ideals. Rather, it consists in a sort of religion of science leading to a straightforward obscurantism through denying what in human beings is connected to the psychical, the spiritual, or the imaginary and fantasy. Whence a blindness with regard to the irrational departures of scientific discourse. There is a good illustration of this attitude in the dialogue of 1998 that pitted Changeux against Ricoeur.

In the course of the discussion, Changeux criticizes Protestant supporters of creationism. After having replaced Darwinian theory with the biblical account of Genesis, they had succeeded in the 1980s in getting the teaching of evolution banned in a number of universities in the United States. In his argument, Changeux contrasts religion and science in an unbelievably simplistic way. In his eyes, religion is always to be suspected of reactionary departures and science always invested with a pure ideal of progress. Without getting flustered, Ricoeur then gets him to notice that the paradox in this business is that the creationists have received the support of numerous scientists, whereas well-known theologians have taken up the defense of evolutionism.[4]

The difference between the French and American situations of psychoanalysis is not to be explained by mind-sets or by local characteristics but rather by geopsychoanalysis,[5] in other words, by the dynamic of modes of implantation of Freudianism specific to each region of the world. In this regard, it should not be forgotten that France is the only country in the world where, for a whole century, the necessary conditions came together for a successful integration of psychoanalysis into every sector of cultural life, via both psychiatric and intellectual routes. So in this domain France is an exception. It is not because of some national superiority but because of a particular experience.

Linked to a major event in human history, this exceptionality could theoretically be universalized. And indeed this is why it has been able to serve as a model for the institutionalization of democratic principles in numerous countries. Its origin goes back to the Revolution of 1789, which granted scientific and juridical legitimacy to reason's consideration of madness, and then to the Dreyfus affair, which made possible the birth of a self-consciousness on the part of the intelligentsia. Without the 1789 Revolution, there would not have been a body of psychiatric knowledge in France capable of integrating the universal nature of the Freudian discovery, and without the Dreyfus affair, there would not have existed an intellectual avant-garde capable of supporting a subversive representation of the Freudian notion of the unconscious.[6]

In this connection, it is not clear that Hannah Arendt was right when in 1963 she valorized the American model of revolution against the French one, stressing that the first rested on an ethics of freedom, whereas the second privileged the primacy of equality.[7] Even if French egalitarianism did result in the Terror, provisionally relinquishing the establishment of liberty in favor of the collective happiness of the people,[8] it is acknowledged today that the famous American model of the primacy of liberty is seriously troubled, by puritanism and liberalism as much as by scientism or communitarianism. On the other hand, it does seem that the French model, relieved of egalitarianism, is more the bearer of an ideal of liberty.

It is this French exceptionality that embarrasses both those who advocate the abolition of the revolutionary ideal and those in favor of behavior-modification man. Both groups la-ment the notorious French "belatedness," hoping that one day the science of the brain will finally manage to finish off the supposed archaisms of Freudian doctrine, even if it means resuscitating the ancient conceptions of the unconscious (cerebral, hereditary, or automatic). This lamentation bespeaks the secret hope that the ancient figure of the intellectual—Socratic sage, visionary poet, or politically involved philosopher—might one day be replaced by that of the specialist or the expert with the job of marking out the infinite platitude of a world reduced to the observable.

It is quite possible, moreover, that this exceptionality is in the process of yielding at the very moment when Freudian universalism, of which it is the bearer, is dissolving into the particularities of different schools of thought. And no doubt, in order to revive it, a new Enlightenment Europe will have to be reconstituted.

⊖

PART III

The Future of Psychoanalysis

CHAPTER 9

Science and Psychoanalysis

Scientists have always considered psychoanalysis to be a hermeneutics. Far from constructing a model of human behavior, Freudian doctrine, if you believe them, is no more than a literary system for interpreting affects and desires. So the right thing to do would be either to exclude it from the field of science along with other disciplines not based on experimentation or to rethink the organization of all these domains (anthropology, sociology, history, linguistics, etc.) in terms of a "cognitive science," the only one able to get them admitted into the category of "real science."

This scientistic approach assumes that there exists a radical separation between the so-called exact sciences and the so-called human sciences. The first are said to be based on the rejection of the irrational and the production of concrete proofs and tangible results, whereas what the second have in common, quite differently, is that they can neither refute the hypotheses they put forward nor make concrete the results they interpret as proofs of the validity of a process of reasoning.

This conception of science leads to some aberrations. Witness, if need be, in the field that interests us, the story of the celebration of the centenary of psychoanalysis that followed the Masson affair.

In December 1995, when a major Freud exhibition, which had been planned for a long time, was being organized at the

Library of Congress in Washington, D.C., a petition signed by forty-two independent researchers, mostly American, was sent to James Billington, director of the library, Michael Roth, chief organizer of the exhibition, and James Hutson, in charge of the manuscripts department. The signatories, including some excellent authors (Phyllis Grosskurth, Elke Mühlleitner, Johannes Reichmayr, Nathan Hale, and others) criticized the future catalog for being too "institutional" and demanded that their own work should appear in it.[1]

To lend support to this collective effort, two of the petition's organizers whose fanaticism is already familiar to us, Peter Swales and Adolf Grünbaum, set in motion a vicious press campaign against Freud, accusing him of sexually abusing his sister-in-law and being guilty of charlatanism.

Frightened by this witch-hunt, the organizers of the exhibition chose to postpone it, even though many American journalists and intellectuals showed their hostility to these extremist stands in the press. It should be said that several exhibitions had already been canceled for similar reasons. One of these, on how slaves lived on the old plantations, had been deemed shocking by the black employees of the Library of Congress, anxious to remove the traces of a past described as humiliating. The exhibition was modified and transferred to the Martin Luther King Library. Another exhibition, on the *Enola Gay*, organized by the Smithsonian, had given rise to a chorus of protest because some air force veterans found it too sympathetic to the victims of Hiroshima. It had to be reconceived around the idea that the bomb was a necessary evil.

This was the context in which another petition was organized in France, on the initiative of Philippe Garnier, a French psychiatrist and psychoanalyst. It criticized both the prying "ayatollahs" and the organizers of the Library of Congress for being incapable of imposing their authority. Signed by a hundred and eighty intellectuals or practitioners from every country, every tendency, and every nationality, this second petition was extremely influential.[2] It put the accent on the puritanical, communitarian, and persecutory madness that was threatening to take over the United States and inciting pressure groups to exercise censorship of the big cultural institutions.

The result of Grünbaum and Swales's anti-Freud offensive was to marginalize the other signatories and favor academicism. The exhibition opened in October 1998 and presented a Freud whose theories no longer had any importance with regard to science and truth. "It hardly matters to me whether Freud's ideas are true or false," Michael Roth insisted. "The important thing is that they have impregnated our whole culture and the way we understand the world through films, art, cartoons, or TV."[3]

So, at the end of the twentieth century and in the name of an arbitrary split established between science and culture, the centenary of psychoanalysis was being commemorated by exhibiting in Washington a Freud without smell or savor and limited to the works of mostly (90 percent) anglophone historians. In short, a perfectly correct Freud, conforming to the canons of the depressive society, was being fabricated with full documentation.[4]

The same period saw a violent challenge to the supposed impostures perpetrated by the language of the human sciences.

In 1996 Alan Sokal, an American physicist with a desire to do battle with the jargon of the so-called postmodern theoretical trend, wrote up with full documentation a text putting in question the most generally accepted scientific truths in the name of a critique of Western metaphysics. After succeeding in getting his article published in the journal *Social Text*, which was connected with this trend, he revealed to the press and interested people that it was a hoax designed to unmask the relativism of these so-called human sciences, daring to utilize the concepts of hard science without understanding anything about them.[5] The story caused a scandal. With the confidence his triumph had given him, Sokal published in France a work cowritten by Jean Bricmont, a Belgian physicist, in which he treated a number of French authors as impostors: Jacques Lacan, Gilles Deleuze, Félix Guattari, Michel Serres, and others.[6]

The interesting thing about this book is that while they are opposing a supposedly rational scientific discourse to relativism, the two scholars fabricate a jargon as incomprehensible as the one they are thrashing.

In an eighteen-page hatchet job that takes up the first chapter, Lacan, in particular, even more than the other thinkers, is accused of talking about theories he doesn't know, of fraudulently importing scientific notions, of showing a superficial erudition and wallowing in the manipulation of meaningless sentences.

To bolster their demonstration, Sokal and Bricmont make use of a manifestly problematic text. This is the famous lecture given in October 1966, at the big symposium organized by Richard Macksey, Eugenio Donato, and René Girard at the Johns Hopkins Humanities Center, with participants such as Lucien Goldmann, Jacques Derrida, Tzvetan Todorov, and Jean-Pierre Vernant. For this structuralist jamboree, where the best French and American academics met together for the first time, Lacan, who was distressed at having to face a new public, had "composed" a text of his own devising. Not speaking English, he had taken it into his head to write (and above all to declaim) his lecture in the language of Shakespeare. A young philosopher, Anthony Wilden, who would soon be letting out a cry of pain right in the middle of the symposium, had been assigned to him as his assistant: his job was to "translate" the speech of an anxious lecturer alternating between French and "English." In 1970 this strange lecture was reprinted (in English) in the proceedings of the Baltimore conference, in the form of a paraphrase of what the speaker had said in two languages. It has a ludicrous title: "Of Structure as an Inmixing of an Otherness Prerequisite to Any Subject Whatever."[7] No one knows the original French text of this lecture, and no serious researchers refer to it today. It does however contain a few fine reflections on time, death, and the spectacle of Baltimore in the early morning. The discussion that follows [in the conference proceedings] is remarkable: those who question Lacan criticize him harshly— not on his lecture, but on his oeuvre, and particularly on the way he uses logic and mathematics.

In their book, Sokal and Bricmont give this lecture an exemplary value. Regarding the published text as indicative of Lacan's approach (and thus his "imposture"), [in the 1997 French edition] they (re)translate it from English to French and cite it at length, six times, with extended quotations. They then declare [in the French text] that in this text Lacan elaborates "his theses on topology for the first time in public."[8] Gross error: too busy tracking down imposture, the two authors are incapable of choosing from or of contextualizing an oeuvre that they are incapable of either reading or criticizing.

Not only was Lacan interested in topology as far back as 1950, but it was in 1965, in his lecture "La science et la vérité"[9] [Science and truth], and not in Baltimore, that he changed his orientation, revealing for the first time in a new way some advances that can be characterized as topological.

After granting far too large a place to an aberrant text arising from an unlikely lecture, Sokal and Bricmont pursue their error—hunting by retranslating a fragment (on *Hamlet*) of a 1959 seminar back into French from English.[10] Knowing nothing about Lacan's oeuvre, they mistakenly claim that the French version does not exist: clearly they do not know the typewritten versions. In their bibliography, moreover, they give the English title incorrectly.

In these circumstances, Sokal and Bricmont are incapable of evaluating Lacan's turn to topology and mathematics; they miss the real impasses and the true genius of Lacan by pointing out mistakes in false texts and then rereading a few fragments of actual texts in the light of an assumed imposture. Their conclusion from this is that the impostor is the prophet of a "lay mysticism" or, better, the founder of a new religion. Reading a work like this, where both the manipulation of texts and ignorance of them authorize the fabrication of imaginary impostures, one is justified in asking who is the real impostor.

Against these scientistic discourses fostering the worst excesses of detective-style normalization, we must set a quite different figure of science: not Science conceived as a dogmatic abstraction, taking the place of god or a repressive theology, but sciences in the plural, organized with rigor, anchored in a history, and divided according to the modes of knowledge production. Since Galileo, science has been defined as knowledge of the laws governing natural processes; it has since given rise to many approaches, whose point in common is that they all remove the analysis of human reality from the ancient domination of the so-called divine sciences, based on revelation. Whence the existence, from the end of the eighteenth century, of a plurality of domains, leading to different types of knowledge that can be classified in three branches: the formal sciences (logic and mathematics), the natural sciences (physics, biology), and the human sciences (sociology, anthropology, history, psychology, linguistics, psychoanalysis).[11]

While the formal sciences are based on pure speculation, the natural sciences have both formal and experimental components. The formal sciences discover their object by constructing it, whereas the natural sciences refer to an external object corresponding to empirical data. The human sciences, meanwhile, differ from the other two by setting themselves the task of understanding individual and group behavior starting from three fundamental categories: subjectivity, the symbolic, meaning.

However, as I have shown in relation to the debate on the brain and thought, the human sciences oscillate between two attitudes. One aims at eliminating subjectivity, meaning, or the symbolic in any form and taking physico-chemical, biological, or cognitive processes as its sole model of human reality; the other, in contrast, eagerly claims the importance of these three categories, thinking of them as universal structures. On one side, human beings are approached as machines; on the other, a study of human complexity takes into account the biological body and subjective behavior, whether

in terms of intentionality or lived experience (phenome-
nology), or else via an interpretive theory of symbolic processes (psychoanalysis, anthropology), postulating unconscious mechanisms that function without the subject being
aware of them.

This distinction between natural sciences and human sciences does not mean that the division between the two is im-
permeable. So for instance, the natural sciences are often
concerned with individual questions, while the human sciences can appeal to formal and experimental components
present in the two other branches of science. Furthermore, as
we have seen in relation to mythologies of the brain, no science is out of reach of the tendencies that characterize the irrational approach.

In a recent book, Gilles Gaston Granger brings out very
clearly the three modalities of irrationality peculiar to the history of the sciences.[12] The first appears when a scientist has
to face the obstacle constituted by a set of doctrines governing the thought of a period that have become dogmatic, restrictive, or sterile. What he or she then has to do is innovate,
calling into question a dominant model by summoning up
unusual themes or placing objects in a different light under
science's gaze. For example, the unconscious, madness, unreason, the feminine, the sacred—in short, everything that
Georges Bataille calls the heterogeneous or the accursed
share. Turning to the irrational then makes it possible to re-
suscitate a figure of reason and set off again to conquer another rationality.

The second modality appears when a form of thinking gets
fixed in a dogma or in too restrictive a rationalism. It then
has to move forward against itself, with a view to reaching

more convincing results. Far from rejecting rationality, the thinking prolongs the creative act that had given rise to it by inspiring it with a new vigor.

The third modality involves scientists or creators adopting a mode of thought that is consciously outside rationality. What we see then is people taking to false sciences and to attitudes of systematic rejection of the dominant knowledge. Whence the valorization of magic and religion, associated with a belief in the beyond or the power of an uncontrolled ego.

These three modalities of irrationality can be found in all the sciences and are therefore present in the history of psychoanalysis. Freud, however, always kept within the limits of the first two.

The first moment is marked by the abandonment of the seduction theory. Between 1887 and 1900 Freud constructs a new doctrine of sexuality. In his relationship with Fliess, he then encounters a biological irrationality and adopts the most outlandish theories of his time before imposing the framework of another rationality.

In a second period, from 1920 to 1935, with his doctrine established, he introduces doubt into the heart of psychoanalytic rationality in order to combat the positivism that is threatening it from within. This second modality of the irrational first appears in the hypothesis of the death drive, which totally transforms his system of thought, then in the form of a debate about telepathy.[13] So Freud goes through a stage of speculative irrationality that will subsequently lead him to other innovations.

The notion of the death drive makes it possible to give a clinical explanation as to why a subject unconsciously and repeatedly places him- or herself in painful, extreme, or traumatic situations that revive for him previously lived experiences. But from the anthropological point of view, it also serves to define the essence of civilization's discontents, with civilization permanently confronted by the principles of its own destruction. Crime, barbarity, genocide are acts that form part of humanity itself, of what is specific to mankind. Since they are inscribed at the heart of the human race, they cannot be excluded from either the particular functioning of each subject or the social collectivity, even in the name of a supposed animal nature external to humanity. Bertolt Brecht's famous "monstrous beast" derives not from animality but from human beings themselves inhabited only by the force of the death drive, the most blind, compulsive, and invasive.

To put this another way, Eichmann in Jerusalem is not an inhuman monster but a subject whose normality is close to madness. Whence the fear one feels hearing him say that he condemns the Nazi system even as he protests the validity of his oath of loyalty to that same system that made him the conscious and servile instrument of an abominable crime.[14] Watching the footage of the trial, you can see that the banality of evil does exist, as Hannah Arendt maintains;[15] it expresses not an ordinary form of behavior but a murderous madness characterized by an excess of normality. Nothing is closer to pathology than the cult of normality pushed to the limit. As we well know, the maddest, most criminal, most deviant forms of behavior often emerge from the most apparently normal of families.

In this connection, Freudian concepts make it possible to grasp the logic of an Eichmann much better than Arendt does.[16] In the same way that not just anyone goes mad, so not just anyone becomes an exterminator, as Claude Lanzmann rightly insists: "Eichmann was definitely not a minor official. His anti-Jewish zeal knew no bounds. He was perfectly well aware that he was committing an enormous crime. One can always say that evil is banal, that nothing is more banal than trains for transporting victims. But those who organized and those who carried out the crime were conscious of the extraordinary nature of what they were perpetrating."[17]

Eichmann's madness is in the image of Nazi thought, which utilizes science as a delirium, even as it makes it look absolutely normal. In the Nazi universe, everything seems coherent, correct, logical, clean, well-ordered, rational. In the name of the most elaborate science and with the help of the most modern of technologies, an inversion of the norm was established, in the service of a genocide, the most formidable imaginable, since this inversion itself becomes the figure of the norm. Never mind if the norm is cut off from any reference to a symbolic order, for in this kind of universe the essential thing is that the abolition of reason has become the norm. This logic explains the "torments" of Eichmann and his masters in extermination: in 1944 they were much more anxious to rationalize the process of annihilating the Jews than to win the war against the Allies.[18]

This is the drive to destruction, accentuated by the technological mastery of the forces of nature, that Freud is referring to in 1929 when he writes the final prophetic sentences of his book *Civilization and Its Discontents*: "Men have gained control over the forces of nature to such an extent that with their help they would have no difficulty in exterminating one another to the last man. They know this, and hence comes a large part of their current unrest, their unhappiness and their mood of anxiety."[19]

In the history of psychoanalysis and its origins, telepathy gets put into the category of phenomena derived from occultism, in other words from that neospiritualist movement bringing together miracle workers, philosophers, magi, and mystics that appeared at the end of the nineteenth century as a reaction against the positivism of the forms of knowledge taught in Western universities. This was an attempt to bring together themes shared by Western and Eastern religions in a popular syncretism propagated by different sects. The objective of the movement was the rehabilitation of forms of knowledge called occult or repressed by so-called official science as well as by religions institutionalized into churches.

Yet if psychoanalysis was formed in rupture with official forms of knowledge, it draws its force not from a revalorization of these occult and repressed knowledges but from the rational understanding of previously marginalized phenomena such as dreams. For this reason, we can see why Freud became passionately interested in telepathy.[20] It constitutes a sort of remainder that escapes science, and on this subject Freud is sometimes in dialogue with Ferenczi, sometimes with Jones. Against the former, who is a hard-and-fast believer in the existence of thought transmission, he is constantly changing his opinion, ending up by interpreting the phenomenon with the tools of psychoanalysis; he calls it "transfer of thought" and claims to explain it rationally. In relation to Jones, who is asking him to give up his penchant for occultism to save psychoanalysis doctrine from the accusation of charlatanism, he insists on his refusal to see psychoanalysis shut up in an approach that is too positivistic.

All these oscillations show that Freud only subscribes to the first two models of irrationality. For there is in his doctrine an original pact linking psychoanalysis to Enlightenment philosophy and thus to a definition of a subject founded on reason.

Very different from this approach, the third modality of irrationality makes its appearance in the history of psychoanalysis, even in Freud's lifetime, at the point where it returns to practices that deny both the power of the founding pact and the deconstruction of that pact. This phenomenon is manifest today in certain schools of psychoanalysis that have given up on the very idea of a rational explanation of the mind.

If we keep to the preceding descriptions, it appears that psychoanalysis is indeed a science of humanity. And if Freud was permanently tempted to integrate it into the natural sciences, he never took the plunge and in the end elaborated a more speculative model that could take account of concepts that were not directly linked to clinical experience. He called this model metapsychology, alluding to metaphysics, the branch of philosophy that deals with speculative things, with being or the immortality of the soul. This metapsychology took in, among others, the unconscious, the drives, repression, narcissism, the ego, and the id.

It is through metapsychology that the new doctrine of the unconscious breaks with classical psychology. So instead of blaming Freud for having let go of science or for not having understood a thing about philosophy, wouldn't it be more appropriate to understand the way that he translates metaphysics into a metapsychology and invents an interpretive system making it possible to deconstruct[21] the founding myths of monotheistic religion and Western society? "One could venture to explain in this way the myths of paradise and the fall of man, of God, of good and evil, of immortality, and so on, and to transform *metaphysics* into *metapsychology*."[22] A whole program.

CHAPTER 10

Tragic Man

Psychoanalysis acquires its specific status through its meta-psychological ambition. This is what makes it possible to oppose tragic man, real crucible of modern consciousness, to behavior-modification man, feeble scientistic creature invented by the supporters of the brain-as-machine. Against the nameless monster fabricated by a megalomanic scientist, psychoanalysis sets the destiny of Victor Frankenstein, meaning the trajectory of a subject shot through with his dreams and utopias but limited in his murderous passions by the sanction of the law.

The structure of this tragic man can be found in Oedipus and Hamlet. Just as Sophocles' king endures his destiny like a curse that makes him other than himself, so Shakespeare's prince internalizes it as a repetitive figure of the same. Tragedy of revelation on one side, drama of repression on the other. "As ancient hero, Oedipus symbolizes the universality of the unconscious disguised as destiny; as modern hero, Hamlet refers to the birth of a guilty subjectivity, during a period in which the traditional image of the Cosmos is coming undone," writes Jean Starobinski.[1]

If Freud had remained dependent on a neurophysiological model, he would never have been able to bring the great myths of literature alive to construct a theory of human behavior. In other words, without the Freudian reinterpretation of the founding myths, Oedipus would be only a fictional character and not a universal model of psychical functioning: there would be no Oedipus complex and no oedipal organization of the Western family. Similarly, if Freud had not invented the death drive, we would probably be deprived of a tragic representation of the historic questions that modern consciousness has to face up to. As for psychology, it would have got lost in the hedonistic cult of the power of identity, promoting a smooth, faultless subject entirely shut up in a physico-chemical model.

One of the main arguments leveled against the Freudian system, in particular by Karl Popper and his heirs, is its non-falsifiable, unverifiable, or irrefutable nature. Unable to put its own foundations in question, psychoanalysis does not fit the criteria that would let it enter the world of the sciences.[2] This analysis is seductive but reductive. It depends, in fact, on the hypothesis that there is an irreducible opposition between science over here and pseudo-sciences over there. Now this division does not take account either of the links joining science and scientism, or of irrational offshoots, or of the status of the rational forms of knowledge whose methods are related to those of science, or of the inclusion of subjectivity in the field of the human sciences. In other words, to understand what rationality in psychoanalysis might be, we have to get away from this hypothesis and show that the criterion for the scientificity of a theory depends as much on its ability to invent new explanatory models as on its permanent capacity to reinterpret the old models according to acquired experience.

Freud never stopped reworking his own concepts. Not only did he modify his theory of sexuality according to his clinical experience—particularly in relation to women—but he also completely transformed his doctrine, by moving from the first topic (conscious, unconscious, preconscious) to the second (ego, id, superego) and then by forging the notion of the death drive. What is more, as a system of thought, psychoanalysis gave rise to theoretical trends that were distinct from one another and expressed important reworkings.

Freudianism includes the whole set of trends[3] claiming to derive at once from a clinical method centered on the talking cure (psychoanalysis) and from a theory assuming a shared reference to sexuality, the unconscious, and the transference. But the divergences between tendencies are crucially important. They show how the history of psychoanalysis is confused with that of the successive interpretations that have been made of the original doctrine constructed by Freud. And it is precisely because it has given rise to all these components that Freudianism has produced both a dogmatism and the conditions for a critique of this dogmatism: an official historiography based on the idealization of its own origins (idolatry of the founding master) and a scholarly historiography capable of revising this dogmatism. Finally, like all scientific innovations, it has aroused resistances, conflicts, hatreds, and revisionary attitudes. The fiercest anti-Freudianism—from Grünbaum to Swales—is also a product of Freudianism.

Classical Freudianism—as elaborated in Vienna by Freud—thus depends on the double model of Oedipus and Hamlet: the unconscious tragedy of incest and crime is repeated in the drama of the guilty conscience. At the heart of this configuration, Freud gives a fundamental place to patriarchy. But he knows it is in decline. So his theory of the oedipal family, as he shows in 1912 in *Totem and Taboo*, depends on the idea of a possible symbolic revalorization of an irremediably dethroned paternity. For Freud, the father, like Wagner's Wotan, is a figure who has been abolished, smashed, crushed by the mounting power of female emancipation.

Unlike Bachofen or Weininger, Freud is never antifeminist. Far from setting the past against the present, or "good patriarchy" against the dangers to come of a so-called matriarchal feminization of the body social, he makes the defeat of paternal tyranny into a necessary condition of the coming of democratic societies. And to illustrate his thesis, he borrows from Darwin the myth of the primal horde. Here it is in outline: In primitive times, people lived in small hordes, each of them under the despotic sway of a male who appropriated all the females to himself. One day, the sons of the tribe, rebelling against the father, put an end to the reign of the primal horde. In an act of collective violence, they killed the father and ate his corpse. After the murder, however, they felt repentant, disowned their crime, and then invented a new social order by putting in place all at once exogamy, the prohibition of incest, and totemism. That was the model shared by all religions, especially monotheism.

The Oedipus complex, says Freud, is nothing other than the expression of two repressed desires (desire for incest, desire to kill the father) contained in the two taboos that belong to totemism: prohibition of incest, prohibition on killing the father-totem. As a result, it is universal since it expresses the two major founding prohibitions of all the human sciences.

Put another way, Freud brings anthropology two themes: the moral law and guilt. In the place of the origin is a real act: the necessary murder; in the place of the horror of incest, a symbolic act: the internalization of the prohibition. Every society is thus founded on a regicide, but it does not free itself from murderous anarchy unless the murder is followed by sanctions and by a reconciliation with the image of the father.

Totem and Taboo can thus be read more as a political than as an anthropological book. What it proposes is a theory of democratic power centered on three necessities: founding act, institution of the law, relinquishment of despotism.[4]

This classic oedipal model was challenged between the wars by Melanie Klein and the English school. After the Freudian conception of a patriarchal family, where the father was dispossessed of the marks of his tyranny, came the Kleinian vision of a familial organization from which the father was in a way evicted. In 1924 Karl Abraham revised the Freudian theory of stages, introducing the idea that the subject was modeled through its imaginary relations with objects. The way was then open for a radical reversal of the Freudian perspective. Rather than thinking of the evolution of the subject in terms of passing through biological stages, the aim was rather to show how precocious fantasmatic activity was organized according to types of object relations.

In 1934 Melanie Klein recentered the whole of Freudian clinical practice on the objects themselves, lived as good or bad, frustrating or satisfying, persecutory or strengthening, and so on. With this gesture, she moved child psychoanalysis out of the domain of education and adult psychoanalysis out of the field of neurosis. Rather than analyze children with a parent as intermediary, as Freud had done, and instead of refusing to take them for therapy under the age of four, as Anna Freud recommended, Melanie Klein abolished all the barriers prohibiting direct access to the infantile unconscious.

This was how she conceived of the frame necessary for verbal and nonverbal expression of children's psychical activity: toys, animals, balls, marbles, pencils, modeling clay, small-scale furniture, and so on.

If Freud was the first to discover the repressed child in the adult, Melanie Klein was the first to reveal what was already repressed in the child: the infant. Studying the archaic relationship to the mother then makes it possible to gain a better grasp of the origin of psychoses, which generally derive from a destructive fusion with the maternal body, experienced as a persecuting object. Against the classic oedipal model, the Kleinians thus set up a preoedipal model, going back to a distressing universe of strong symbiosis with the mother: a primitive world, inaccessible to the law, no longer given over to paternal despotism but to the cruelty of maternal chaos. The successor to the figure of Freudian tragic man, prey to neurotic conflict and the need for a reconciliation with his guilty conscience, was thus the vision of Kleinian tragic man: a subject on the borderline of madness and devoured from within by his or her own fantasies before even having been able to enter into conflict with the world.

The theoretical and clinical battle that from 1934 set the classic Freudians against the Kleinians is closely related to the quarrel of the Ancients and the Moderns. The backcloth to the oedipal model invented by Freud was fin-de-siècle Viennese society, tormented by its own agony, by its shameful sensuality, and by the cult of atemporality.[5] Not only were fathers losing their authority just as the Hapsburg monarchy was foundering under the weight of its arrogance, but women's bodies seemed threatened by a forceful desire for pleasure. And this inclination had every chance of abolishing the ancient order, heavily immobile, and promoting the institution of the modern state where the place of the father, as a symbol of unity, would gradually disappear. Engendered by the decline of this paternal function, psychoanalysis was trying with Freud to revalorize the dethroned father symbolically via a new theory of the family centered on the figure of Oedipus. Far from being backward-looking, this theory enabled the subject, closed in on his or her private life, to free herself from the ancient hierarchy and accede to liberty.

The setting for Klein's reworking, by contrast, was interwar English society, whose ideals it reflected. In this democratic world, where the emancipation of women was further advanced than in Vienna, reflecting on the omnipresent place of the mother in children's education seemed more important than the Viennese attempt to restore a hypothetical paternal function, even at the cost of a symbolization.

From this point of view, the Kleinian model was more "modern" than Freud's and had more of a grasp on the problems raised by the evolution of Western society in the second half of the twentieth century. So it made considerable headway in the psychoanalytic movement, becoming the main point of reference for the IPA (International Psychoanalytic Association), both in Europe (except for France) and in Latin American countries. In the wake of Kleinianism, the British school further extended its influence across the entire world through the quality of its chief representatives' clinical writings, especially D. W. Winnicott's.

Kleinianism was tipping psychoanalytic theory as a whole toward the child battling it out with maternal power, but the theses of self psychology, which essentially developed in the United States, also required a revision of classic Freudianism.

We owe the finest elaboration of these theses, of which traces can be found in a number of other components of Freudianism, to Heinz Kohut, an American psychoanalyst of Viennese origin. Kohut was a member of the IPA but rebelled against the conservatism of psychoanalytic dignitaries who shut up analysis in a fixed ritual. Kohut sought to breathe new life into an American Freudianism bogged down in pragmatism and dogma.

Heir to both the Viennese tendency and the Kleinian reworking, Kohut invented a third way that consisted of thinking about disorders of subjectivity in terms of problems of relating linked to social changes. He saw the self as having become the object of every kind of narcissistic investment in a world where the collapse of the great patriarchal values was leading to the idealization of a figure of individuality immersed in the contemplation of his own image. Whence the idea that the myth of Narcissus was better adapted than that of Oedipus to take account of civilization's new discontents.

Kohut notes that the archaic deficiency of the subject can be imputed to a lack of maternal affection that renders him or her unable to maintain a relationship with another. Feeling empty, he masks his mutilation beneath the exterior of a "fake" ego (a self).[6] For Kohut, the subject reconstructs a "grandiose self" structured by an idealized parental imago.[7] From this perspective, Hamlet becomes a narcissistic hero whose weakened self holds out no resistance to the tragedies of a society that has lost all its bearings.

This movement from Oedipus to Narcissus well demonstrates how 1960s psychoanalysis attempted to solve the problems of a subjectivity given over to individualism and chemical substances. Reduced to reflecting himself in the infinite unhappiness of his image, the tragic man of this self psychoanalysis was the ultimate expression of a care for the self that would soon fall into the nothingness of a society converted to the paradigm of depression.

After assimilating the Kleinian reworking, Jacques Lacan, too, proposed a revision of the classic oedipal model. From 1938, in a celebrated article on family complexes, he was painting a somber picture of the universe of the Western family, which he saw as shot through with every form of social disgrace, every form of subjective violence, every form of conformity. The theme of the sacred and the antibourgeois nihilism that animated his pen did not prevent him from being skeptical with regard to the October Revolution. So he judged the Communist attempts to abolish the family as wicked. They were utopian and, he thought, risked leading to a more serious authoritarianism than the one imposed by familial legitimacy.

After the war, Lacan therefore upheld the values of an enlightened conservatism, indebted to Tocqueville. But he also made use of the theses of Georges Bataille and Marcel Mauss, while advocating the cult of a subversive Freudianism as the only means for thinking about the social bond, the imaginary, the sacred, the subject.

In this regard, Lacan was more Freudian than the Kleinians and the partisans of self psychoanalysis. He did after all draw on the classic oedipal thesis in order to give a new value to the paternal function. Subsequently, it was through reading Claude Lévi-Strauss's *Elementary Structures of Kinship* that he discovered the theoretical tool that enabled him to conceptualize this function in structural terms.[8] Using the principles of Saussurian linguistics, he made language the condition of the unconscious, dropping the Freudian idea of the biological substratum, inherited from Darwinism. From this perspective he definitively elaborated his new topic (symbolic, imaginary, real) and his theory of naming. Thus it was that the dispossessed, humiliated, defeated father haunting Western consciousness at the end of the nineteenth century reappeared with Lacan as invested with a linguistic power. He was in a sense reconstructed in the concept of the Name-of-the-Father[9] and restricted to a power of nomination, even as he was disintegrating in the social reality of the new forms of family organization.

Lacan was without question the greatest theorist of Freudianism of the second half of the twentieth century. His conception of tragic man was directly derived from that of the Frankfurt School. First from Kojève, then from Adorno and Horkheimer,[10] he borrowed the themes of the critique of Enlightenment and the negativity of history. So he brought psychoanalysis a breath of the German philosophical tradition. Via this crossover, a subversive act that Freud would never have dreamed of occurred on French soil. For Freud had built his theory on a biological model, refusing to take account of philosophical discourse.

By reinterpreting the oedipal model in the light of structural anthropology, Lacan, as has been said, made paternity into a symbolic construction. As such, and not in virtue of some natural essence, paternity for him was as universal as the family.

On this point, Lacan joined Lévi-Strauss, who in 1956 wrote:

Family life appears practically everywhere in human societies, even in those whose sexual and educational customs are very distant from our own. After having claimed for about fifty years that the family, as modern societies know it, could only be a recent development, the result of a long, slow process of evolution, anthropologists now tend towards the opposite conviction, namely that the family, based on the more or less lasting and socially approved union of a man and a woman, is a universal phenomenon, present in every type of society.[11]

The elaboration of different models of psychical organization clearly shows that the psychoanalytic conception of the family and sexual identity evolves according to transformations in Western society.

After seeking to account for a classic triangulation in which the father, already weakening, nonetheless occupied a dominant place, the Freudian model was then revised by Melanie Klein, who gave the maternal position a decisive place. What the Lacanian perspective did was to make this reign eternal by attributing infinite power to the woman. Her pleasure, for Lacan, makes her "without limits," and through motherhood she wields an awesome power over the child and the father. Lacanian theory thus reflected the ideal that women, having reached an infinite degree of freedom, can decide for themselves about reproductive choice, thanks to contraception, with or without men's agreement. Whence this uncontrollable power that enables her to take away the father's right to appropriate the process of filiation.

Commenting in 1957 on the case of an American woman who, with her husband's frozen sperm, had made use of

postmortem artificial insemination, Lacan had further fore-
seen that maternal omnipotence might one day become a
fetish:

> I leave it to you to extrapolate—from the moment we start
> down this road, then hundreds of years from now we will
> be giving women children who will be the direct sons of
> men of genius living now, and will have been carefully con-
> served in little pots between now and then. The father has
> had something cut off in this event, and in the most radi-
> cal way—as well as his speech. So then the question be-
> comes one of knowing how, by what method, in what
> mode, the ancestor's words will be registered in the child's
> psyche, when the mother is the ancestor's only representa-
> tive and only means of conveyance. How will she get the
> potted ancestor to speak?[12]

As a universal model, the family is an indestructible entity,
being a concrete realization of the structures of kinship—in
other words, of alliance and filiation. It is the source of normality but also, as we know from psychoanalysis, the starting point of every form of psychical pathology: psychoses,
perversions, neuroses, and so forth. So there is no reason to
worry about its future, as do moralists and representatives of
the various religions who regularly express the fear that it
will be destroyed by the spread of divorce. The various
modes of free union and a reconfigured family show, moreover, that this model is perpetuated under forms that are always being renewed. Its force of attraction can be gauged
from the fact that some of those who had been excluded because it was impossible for them to marry (homosexuals)

now want to be included, so as to be able to adopt children. I support the idea that homosexuals should have the same rights as heterosexuals in all domains, but it is only at the point when these rights have been acquired that we can begin to reflect critically on possible new relationships between what is socially regarded as normal and what is socially regarded as abnormal.

Psychoanalysis must always offer its help in struggles against all forms of discrimination—anti-Semitism, homophobia, racism, and any other kind of persecution—because it is the very condition of its own existence. As a discipline, it has always itself been persecuted with the type of argument used against minorities. We should not confuse the discipline with positions adopted by individual analysts, who may have extremely varying opinions but do not represent the sovereign power of a discipline. Yet faced with this desire for children on the part of homosexual couples, psychoanalysis today is having great difficulty in offering coherent responses.[13] In fact, as long as homosexuality was regarded as a form of degeneration, the question of integrating it into the norm was not seriously envisaged. But starting from the moment when Freud refused to classify it among the defects, making it a sexual disposition derived from bisexuality, the way was open for all the questionings that are coming up today.

Freud's heirs, particularly Ernest Jones and Anna Freud, did, however, tend to consider that homosexuality was a sexual pathology that could be cured by a well-conducted analysis. Whence the futile attempt to change homosexuals into heterosexuals, which ended in painful defeat. Despite experience, the IPA, following a decision of 1921, has always refused to admit practicing homosexuals officially into the ranks of the groups that it comprises. It has thus got behind in relation to changes in customs and laws and in relation to other psychoanalytic associations (Lacanian ones in particular) that have been rejecting all forms of discrimination for a long time.

If homosexuality is now no longer regarded as a sexual perversion, in part through psychoanalysis, there is every reason to think that other "abnormal" people will not take long to embody the transgressive ideal of tragic man by taking over from those who have already been included in the norm: childless single people (homosexual or heterosexual), zoophiles, "effeminate" male homosexuals, libertines, prostitutes (men or women), transvestites, transsexuals, and so on.[14]

Beyond the legitimate demand of homosexuals to have access to fatherhood or motherhood, we thus have to ask who will be the Charluses[15] and the Oscar Wildes of tomorrow.

CHAPTER 11

Universality, Difference, Exclusion

While the models elaborated by psychoanalysis develop according to the society in which they unfold, they are also out of sync with them. In most countries where psychoanalysis has taken root and in spite of the progress linked to emancipation movements, women, for instance, are still victims of inequalities, treated as inferior, and underrepresented in the highest spheres of political power, particularly in France. What is more, contraception and abortion rights are often ridiculed by moral and religious traditionalists. But in countries where psychoanalysis has not taken root, the situation is worse since women (like homosexuals, for that matter) are not even considered to be full subjects.

I have shown elsewhere that the nonvariable conditions necessary for Freudian ideas and a psychoanalytic movement to take root are, on the one hand, the establishment of psychiatric knowledge, meaning an approach to madness able to conceptualize the notion of mental illness over any idea of divine possession, and, on the other, the existence of state-backed legal rights able to ensure the free transmission of knowledge.[1]

This conceptualization, as is shown by the emergence of the paradigm of hysteria at the end of the nineteenth century, involves a new way of apprehending the female body. In other words, for psychoanalysis to exist and for rationality to dethrone the idea of possession, it is necessary that women become the vehicle of a contestation of the forms of domination impeding their subjectivity. There is always something feminine in the beginning of psychoanalysis, and it is as though the emergence of this femininity were necessary for the achievement of a transformation of universal subjectivity.

It is generally the absence of one of these elements (establishment of a psychiatric form of knowledge and state-backed legal rights) or of both at once, and not "mentalities," that accounts for Freudianism not taking root or disappearing in totalitarian dictatorships (Nazism/Communism) as well as in Islamically influenced parts of the world, still with a tribal form of community organization.

In this context, it should be stressed that military dictatorships did not prevent the expansion of psychoanalysis in Latin America (especially Brazil and Argentina). That is because of the kind of dictatorship, different from the two totalitarian systems that destroyed it in Europe. These "caudillo" regimes have not been "exterminating" ones. They have not eliminated psychoanalysis as a "Jewish science," as happened with Nazism from 1933 to 1944, or as a "bourgeois science," as happened under Communism from 1945 to 1989. These regimes have persecuted opponents and massacred civilian populations, but they have not sought to destroy a science as such.

It is therefore possible to put forward the hypothesis that in order to make psychoanalysis entirely disappear from a region of the world or to prevent it from taking root where it doesn't exist, either it must be eliminated in the way that you eliminate a race, a people, a class, or a plague; or you must perpetuate modes of interpreting the mind that predate the emergence of scientific medicine (witchcraft, traditional forms of medicine, religious control, etc.). In the first case, the eradication is destructive, since one kind of difference is abolished in the name of another; in the second case, though, it is simply regressive: there is an attempt to reduce the human race to a sum total of localities, through an appeal to cultural relativity. Set up as a fetish, difference is then a source of exclusion. And it is this phenomenon of the fetishization of differences that tends to lead to the disappearance of psychoanalysis in countries where all the conditions for a perfectly successful implantation had been present together for a hundred years: in particular, in the United States.

Demonstrating the existence of a sexual identity (gender) detached from organic or physico-chemical reality doesn't prevent the anatomy, the physiology, and the hormonal functioning of men and women from not being identical. Biological difference exists, and we should take account of it, but it is not everything.

Nor does this difference prevent each subject being different (or other) in his or her way of relating to another or to his own identity. Every human being proceeds with a mask on in relation to his fellow humans, since he is shot through with the desire to make himself liked or recognized. So there is an infinity of differences that, taken together, constitute what is universal in the human race.

This is why, in an egalitarian society, the law has to be the same for all subjects whatever the culture, religion, or identity to which they each wish to attach themselves additionally. As to prohibition, meaning the subjective internalization of a symbolic law (the prohibition of incest, for instance), it is absolutely necessary to the functioning of all human societies.

In other words, it is just as mistaken to valorize universalism in the name of a refusal of difference as to reject universalism in the name of an arbitrary valorization of just one difference: anatomy, for instance, but also gender, color of skin, age, identity, and so on. For the whole of humanity it is just as necessary to have abstract principles of reference (concepts, the law, the symbolic, structures, invariants, etc.) as to take account of the concrete reality of concrete existences: sexuality, private life, social situation, poverty, illness, loneliness, madness, mental suffering, and so on.

Yet what we are seeing with the current fetishization of all differences—*DSM IV*, dissociated unconsciouses, multiple personalities, polarized views of sexual trauma, sexual politics based on simplistic categories, psychical subject reduced to a neurone or to an addictive dependency, and so forth—is an offensive whose aim is to replace the double ideal of the universal and the different by a chain of differentiation in which everyone becomes the sacrificial victim of a crime always attributable to another.[2]

Invented in the United States thirty-five years ago, this fetishization of difference has led to a politics of positive discrimination, or affirmative action, which consists of legally putting in place preferential treatment for human groups that are victims of forms of injustice: blacks, Hispanics, women, homosexuals, and others.[3] This politics has been extremely useful in furthering the emancipation of these minorities. It is based, though, on the idea that, in order to make up for inequality, it is appropriate to valorize one difference over another. The application of this principle, which we have seen operating in relation to the controversy over the Library of Congress Freud exhibition, is increasingly contested nowadays, since it works against its own objectives, generous as they are. We can see why: discrimination can never be positive since it always necessitates the existence of *other* victims whose very difference makes them scapegoats.[4]

In European societies, where multiculturalism does not have the same importance as it does in the United States, Australia, or Canada, it is essentially in women's struggles that the demand for equality risks being transformed into a cult of difference, then into the demand for a positive discrimination,[5] and finally into a downright process of serial exclusions.[6] Corresponding to men's exclusion in paternity, moreover, is the insistence on male participation in household tasks or the care of babies. And similarly, the exclusion of the *other* as different is echoed by a strong urge to reinvent categories, typologies, or *patterns* for distinguishing between "good" and "bad" subjects according to a new "folk psychology" of ethnic groups or genders.

The reduction of thought to a mechanism of the brain obviously supports the proliferation of these modes of fetishization: scientism leads to ethnicism as surely as a rigid universalism leads to communitarianism. For nothing is more destructive for a subject than to be reduced to his or her physico-chemical system, and nothing is more humiliating for that same subject than to see his or her personal suffering brought down to the false difference of an ethnic origin.

If serotonin came to be considered the sole cause of suicide, if the sexual act were in the future assimilated to a rape, if the migrant worker on the edge of the city were no longer regarded as anything more than his or her African amulets, and if, lastly, the figure of tragic man were reduced to the mechanical exercise of vital functions, even as *The* Woman, now all powerful, is identified more with her difference than with full subjecthood, then our societies would be on the verge of plunging into a new barbarism, as alarming as the one that Freud denounced in 1927 when he became aware that Western civilization did not have the means of making humanity set limits to its destructive drives: "Whereas we might at first think that its essence lies in controlling nature for the purpose of acquiring wealth and that the dangers which threaten it could be eliminated through a suitable distribution of that wealth among men, it now seems that the emphasis has moved over from the material to the physical. The decisive question is whether . . . it is possible . . . to reconcile men to [the instinctual sacrifices] which must necessarily remain and to provide a compensation for them."[7]

CHAPTER 12

Critique of Psychoanalytic Institutions

Invented by Enlightenment Jews who were heirs to the Haskalah,[1] psychoanalysis aspired from the outset to become a great liberation movement. Its founders, meeting weekly at the Wednesday Psychoanalytic Society, thought that the exploration of the unconscious ought to enable humanity to calm its sufferings. Psychoanalysis was a revolution in personal meaning; ultimately its first vocation was to change mankind by showing [in Arthur Rimbaud's phrase] that "I is another." This was why, very early on, it wanted to equip itself with an institution capable of translating its conception of the world into a politics.

This was further related to the society in which the first Freudians lived: an empire in decline but whose minorities were protected by an imperial authority that brought them together in spite of their differences, while preventing them from joint disintegration. This was the model that Freud and Ferenczi invoked in 1910 to found the IPA. Refusing to be its president, Freud came to embody the Socratic figure of a master without powers of command.[2]

Through the initiatives first of Max Eitingon and then of Ernest Jones, the IPA was transformed between the wars into a centralized organization with rules aimed at standardizing analysis and at keeping from training "wild" or transgressive analysts or ones deemed too charismatic to practice psychoanalysis appropriately. Also banned were so-called incestuous customs: it was forbidden for practitioners to analyze members of their families or to have sexual relationships with their patients.

This professionalization of the job of psychoanalyst, necessary to the worldwide expansion of Freudianism, went together with the effacement of the figure of the master. Not only did the psychoanalytic movement give up having this figure embodied by an exceptional thinker, but it refused any possibility of the leader of a school resembling Freud. The founding father had to remain unique and inimitable.

While this long process of standardization was beneficial to psychoanalysis, its effect was also to transform the IPA into a machine for the manufacture of worthy citizens. The internationalist spirit that had presided over its creation gave way to the globalism that makes it possible for the IPA of today to export its model training practices to every country "keys in hand," in the way that businesses set up their products and factories in foreign parts.

But by cultivating a norm rather than originality, and globalism over internationalism, the psychoanalysis of worthy citizens has deserted the field of political and intellectual debate. It has been unable to take on board either the challenge of science or social changes. Thinking itself untouchable, it has stopped—despite the individual courage of numerous anonymous practitioners—being concerned with social reality, poverty, unemployment, sexual abuse, and the new demands arising from the transformations in the patriarchal family, on the part of homosexuals in particular who, as I have stressed, are still refused the right to become psychoanalysts. In short, this psychoanalysis has withdrawn its interest from the real world and retreated into its fantasies of omnipotence. It has thus abandoned the young practitioners that it had trained itself and who have ended up no longer believing in the value of Freudian institutions. This is why they criticize it with alacrity and try to conceive of new institutions better adapted to the modern world.

This critical capacity is exercised more or less everywhere in the world. But Latin-American countries (Brazil and Argentina in particular) are definitely in the forefront of the renaissance of Freudianism, primarily because of the particular force of the psychology departments established in their universities, places where the teaching of psychoanalysis takes precedence over other disciplines.

As is the case everywhere else, the French psychoanalytic community is going through a difficult period linked to the general crisis of Western societies: economic crisis, crisis of democratic values, social crisis, absence of hope and of illusions. Unemployment, the fall in incomes, the insecurity of jobs and work, the growing strength of physical forms of psychotherapy and drug treatments, faster and cheaper, have led to a loss of confidence in the Freudian method, parallel to the breakup of large institutions inspired by universal ideals. In short, the social and political fabric in which Freudianism had been successfully established since the end of World War II has become less receptive to the clinical practice of psychoanalysis.

As a result, the great republican institutions—schools and mental health organizations (psychiatric hospitals, medical-psychological centers, and so on)—are nowadays subject to economic imperatives that are not very compatible with the longer term required for a Freudian analysis, even as the progressive disintegration of these institutions is leading to uncontrollable situations of violence and delinquency.

In spite of it all, though, the French psychoanalytic community remains solid. In France there is a total of five thousand psychoanalysts, spread over more than twenty associations, which is eighty-six analysts per million: the highest rate in the world, above Argentina and Switzerland. Eight or nine hundred of them (including trainees) belong to the two societies that are members of the IPA: the Société psychanalytique de Paris [Paris Psychoanalytic Society] (SPP) and the Association psychanalytique de France [French Psychoanalytic Association] (APF). Other psychoanalysts are mostly members of groups or associations deriving from the former Ecole freudienne de Paris [Paris Freudian School] founded by Jacques Lacan in 1964 and dissolved during his lifetime in 1980.

Historians of the movement have taken to classifying groups and individuals according to the generation they belong to. They use two methods of cataloging: one is international and deals with members of the Freudian diaspora scattered around the world; the other relates to individual countries and makes it possible to register the transferential filiation of every practitioner (who analyzed whom), starting from a pioneer group (reducible to a single person in some countries).

In France, there have been three generations. The first consists of the founders of the SPP in 1926. Three of them had dominant roles: Marie Bonaparte, René Laforgue, and Rudolph Loewenstein. Through her friendship with Freud, her celebrity, and her constant activity as a translator and a militant devotee of the Freudian cause, Marie Bonaparte was the movement's principal organizer. Opposite her, Laforgue and Loewenstein became the two principal training analysts of the SPP. It was they who trained the second French generation between the wars, in particular those who would be the leaders of the movement after 1945: Daniel Lagache, Jacques Lacan, Françoise Dolto, Sacha Nacht, and Maurice Bouvet.

Then came the third generation, born in the 1920s and trained by the second generation. They had to face up to two splits, the first in 1953, around the question of lay analysis,[3] the second ten years later (1963), when Jacques Lacan was not accepted as a training analyst in the ranks of the IPA because of his refusal to submit to the existing rules for the length of sessions and the training of analysts.[4] Lacan was in fact refusing to comply with the then obligatory fifty-five-minute sessions and proposing to break them off with significant punctuations giving meaning to the patient's words. Further, he criticized the idea of the dissolution of the transference as the end point of the analysis. In his eyes, an analysis was sustained through a transferential relationship that was never finished with. Finally, he refused the principle of a radical separation between a so-called training analysis and a so-called therapeutic (or personal) analysis: this meant that a trainee should be free to choose his or her analyst without having to resort to a list of those authorized and qualified for the purpose. Moreover—and this is presumably the deeper reason for the rupture—through his teaching and his style, Lacan was bringing back the Freudian figure of the Socratic master at a time when this was considered disastrous by the IPA, more concerned with training good psychoanalytic professionals than with reviving the elitist ambitions at the heart of the movement.

The second split, by far the more serious, was a drama, first of all for Lacan himself, who had never imagined leaving Freudian legitimacy behind, but also for the entire third French generation. Its most brilliant members had been analyzed by him and all of a sudden found themselves in opposing camps: one side grouped together in the APF, which was affiliated to the IPA in 1965, the other in the EFP and definitively rejected by the legitimate Freudian authorities, even though they thought of themselves as much more Freudian than their IPA counterparts, now their rivals.

Unlike their American or British colleagues, third-generation French analysts belonging to the IPA never formed a homogeneous school. Nor did the major trends of international Freudian thought ever get established in France: neither ego psychology, nor Kleinianism, nor Anna-Freudianism, nor self psychology, nor the post-Kleinian theories of Wilfred Ruprecht Bion. It has thus been Lacanianism, and nothing but Lacanianism, that has polarized the field of French psychoanalysis for more than thirty years: non-Lacanians (sometimes known as "orthodox Freudians") on one side and Lacanians on the other, with everyone of course claiming descent from Freud.

This polarization of French Freudianism was accentuated by the presence of Françoise Dolto in the ranks of the EFP. Dolto had a remarkable flair for clinical work; she was the founder of child analysis in France, a figure equivalent to that of Melanie Klein for British psychoanalysis, although her own ideas were closer to Anna Freud's views. Now in 1963, at the time of the second split, Dolto, was not accepted into the IPA. The reasons given to justify this refusal were the opposite of the ones put forward against Lacan: objection was made not to short sessions (hers were according to the rules) but to training analysis practice that was too charismatic and not, so they said, compatible with the standards of classical training. In fact, Dolto was inheriting the hostility that those in charge of the IPA had always shown toward her analyst, René Laforgue, whose technique and practice were considered deviant, meaning too close to those of a Ferenczi or a Rank.

The upshot of all this was that after 1964 the two principal figures of French psychoanalysis delivered their teaching outside the auspices of the IPA.

The conflicts dividing the third generation had considerable repercussions for the two that followed, born between 1935 and 1950. For fifteen years, they had to put up with the in-fighting and narcissistic wounds of their brilliant senior colleagues. They admired them for their writings and their training skills, but they also saw them constantly tearing themselves apart over an omnipresent master: Jacques Lacan. Condemned for his practice, misrecognized for his doctrine, and demonized by both IPA member associations, Lacan was now starting to be an object of idolatry in his own school. As a result, in each camp the two new generations, the fourth and fifth, inherited a history of conflict. This was bequeathed either by Lacan's fellow travelers, who all too often imitated the master's style, or by his adversaries, who detested him and caricatured his personality.

Whereas the two IPA member associations denounced the Lacanians as non-Freudians, the Lacanians regarded their IPA colleagues as bureaucrats who had betrayed psychoanalysis for a form of adaptive psychology in the service of capitalism triumphant. In short, the first group saw the second as sorcerers' apprentices, adepts of so-called five-minute sessions and incapable of putting in place a serious psychoanalytic framework, while the second group regarded the first as orthodox and deintellectualized, in the service of a so-called American psychoanalysis.

This compartmentalization was burst open at the end of the 1970s when René Major, an SPP training analyst open to Lacanian culture and clinical practice, and Serge Leclaire, faithful Lacanian but giving his services to a vast project, "Freudian Republic," joined forces to enable analysts of the next generations to meet up at last outside their various associations. This was the period of the Confrontation movement that made it possible for analysts from all over to criticize their institutions and exchange their points of view, particularly on the subject of how to practice psychoanalysis. For if the two IPA-affiliated associations were shot through with conflicts over the training of analysts, the EFP was going through a serious crisis as a result of the failure of the *passe* experiment.

In this "passing" procedure, invented by Lacan in 1967 and put in place in 1969, an analysand (or *passant*) wanting to become a training analyst would lay out for colleagues (or *passeurs*) those elements in his or her history and analysis that had led him to want to be an analyst. The *passeurs* in their turn would lay out the motivations of the *passant* to a jury of training analysts, and the jury then took a decision either to elect or to reject the candidate. The aim of the process was to replace the classic system of psychoanalytic training by a real interrogation of the training analyst's status.

It was in this context that Lacan made a remark that gave rise to a lot of commentary: "The psychoanalyst is authorized only by him- or herself."[5] With this sentence, he was indicating that the passage to "being-an-analyst"[6] involves a subjective trial linked to the transference. This gives rise, for both candidate and training analyst, to a situation of loss, castration, even melancholy.

The idea of studying how this well-known passage of initiation actually worked was a remarkable one. But the *passe* process did not have the anticipated effect. It led the EFP to a failure then to dissolution, after provoking a third split in 1969, with the departure of a number of analysts, including François Perrier and Piera Aulagnier. Brought together in a "Fourth Group," they founded the Organisation psychanalytique de langue française [French-Language Psychoanalytic Organization] (OPLF).

The two most recent generations of French psychoanalysts were thus led to think about their institutional future in new terms. Generally speaking, the young Lacanians felt freer in relation to the masters who had trained them than did the members of the two IPA groups. Because of the dissolution of the EFP and the breaking apart of Lacanianism into different currents (post-Lacanian or neo-Lacanian), these later generations created a lot of new associations. Freed from every kind of submissive relationship to the masters of the third generation, they have now gone through the process of mourning the ideal institution by giving up the idea of the School that Lacan wished for in times past.

From another point of view, analysts of the most recent SPP and APF generations carry the weight of the quarrels and disappointments of the old ones more heavily. They are more beholden to the analysts who trained them and who remain in the leading ranks of their associations, very attached to their prerogatives and their privileges. So they are quicker to revolt when a conflict breaks out. Whence the institutional violence, often masked, that runs through the two IPA societies.

Folded in on itself for thirty years, and cultivating its "difference" and aestheticism, the APF has not wished to open its ranks to the numerous "pupils" who follow its teachings and at fifty have practically no hope any more of progressing up its hierarchy. Their disappointment gets translated into a certain mockery of all institutional power.

Scattered among twenty or so associations, former Lacanians are nowadays divided over both practice and analytic training, but this does not prevent them from maintaining friendly relations with one another. If the majority of groups have retained the *passe* process, they have transformed it into a ritual without a great deal of scope. For session lengths, almost all have taken up the idea of punctuation while maintaining the principle of the analysand's free choice of analyst. But none has reduced the session time to five minutes, let alone one minute, as Lacan did during the last five years of his life. This practice is nowadays imitated only by a restricted number of practitioners, who can be counted on the fingers of one hand.

There remains, however, a big difference between the clinical practice of Lacanian Freudians and that of Freudians belonging or connected to the IPA. For the former, the length of sessions is not fixed, whereas for the latter a fixed length remains compulsory and is part of the framework of the analysis: now from forty-five to fifty minutes. And in the two French member groups of the IPA, hierarchies and career paths follow international standards.

It must be acknowledged that there are good and bad practitioners in all the French psychoanalytic groups. For in fact—and this is a new contemporary phenomenon—no one association has the monopoly of good clinical practice any more. They have all been weakened by the splits, the conflicts, the institutional inflexibility; and they have all lost their prestige, so much so that many therapists no longer seek to join them or else have no hesitation in being members of two (or even three) institutions at once.

From 1996 to 1999 the reorganization of the field of psychoanalysis took the form of a double process: a proliferation of splits on one side, federalism on the other. So the Association mondiale de psychoanalyse [World Association of Psychoanalysis] (AMP), created by Jacques-Alain Miller, imploded, giving birth to diverse autonomous movements. Today, centralizing institutions are much less credible than small units, more lively, more creative, and always ready to link up to make it easier to exchange pieces of knowledge and clinical experience with one another. Witness the creation, in Barcelona in October 1998, of a Convergence Movement (Convergencia) linking forty-five Lacanian associations. From a wider perspective, René Major's initiation of the Etats Généraux [States General] of psychoanalysis clearly indicates that Freudianism in the twenty-first century should orient itself toward a new type of collaboration, that of associated networks, responding to the new demands of civil society. No doubt the years to come will also see a serious challenge to the classificatory imperialism of the *DSM* and the cognitive sciences, whose ineffectiveness we are beginning to ponder even while they are at their height.

France has not had to confront the wave of anti-Freudianism that is raging in the United States. Neither Freud nor psychoanalysis is attacked with such virulence in Europe. Even so, despite their undeniable usefulness, the different schools of psychoanalysis are still suffering from a real discredit because of their tendency to dogmatism.

When it comes to contemporary patients, they bear little resemblance to those of earlier periods. Generally speaking, they fit the image of this depressive society in which they live. Impregnated with contemporary nihilism, they present with narcissistic or depressive disturbances and suffer from solitude and symptoms of loss of identity. Often lacking either the energy or the desire to submit to long analyses, they have trouble with regular attendance at analysts' consulting rooms. They often miss sessions and can often no longer stand more than one or two a week. Lacking financial means, they tend to suspend the analysis as soon as they realize there has been an improvement in their condition, even if that means taking it up again when the symptoms reappear. This resistance to entering into the transference setup indicates that if the market economy treats subjects like commodities, patients too have a tendency in their turn to use analysis as a form of medication and the analyst as a receptacle for their sufferings.

The model of the typical analysis, handed down from generation to generation through the mythical image of the armchair and the couch, is now restricted to the privileged. The majority of young therapists no longer practice psychoanalysis full-time, and in place of the classic setup, tend to substitute a face-to-face analytic situation that looks like a psychotherapy. In this connection, it is worth noting that Lacanians are more ready to accept these transformations, steeped as they are in the doctrinal issues of psychoanalysis, whereas their SPP and APF colleagues prefer to give this new situation the name of "analytic psychotherapy" in order to distinguish it more clearly from the classic model of the typical analysis, deemed untouchable.

If the patients have changed, the psychoanalysts of the younger generations don't look like their elders either. In this regard, there are fewer differences than there used to be between the Lacanians and the other Freudians. They have all taken the same psychology courses, and many have another job apart from psychoanalysis (generally they are clinical psychologists). Whatever their affiliations, they have few private patients and mainly work in institutions, where they get other techniques going: drama therapy, family and group psychotherapy. They all have posts in the health services: helping with drug addicts, prostitutes, delinquents, AIDS sufferers, emergency care, and so forth.

Entering the profession via medicine, psychiatry, philosophy, or literary studies is clearly on the wane to the benefit, as I have said, of psychology. And the historical and theoretical culture of the average analyst today is different from what it was in previous generations. More modest than their elders, young practitioners are often keen to acquire a knowledge that their university courses have not given them. This is why so many of them go to the conferences that address the big problems of today: drugs, emigration, violence, the new forms of shared lives and sexuality, death, old age, and so on.

Despite all the difficulties that confront it, this generation seeks a renewal of Freudianism. They are closer than their elders were to social deprivation, which they face on site, and also more pragmatic, more direct, more humanist, more sensitive to all forms of exclusion, and more demanding in their ethical choices. Their courses orient them toward clinical psychology, and they have done with mourning a bygone age in which the figure of the master still embodied the ideals of a subversive and elitist Freudianism. And so they have detached themselves from the conflictual passions that marked the preceding period. Less theoretical and more clinical, they demonstrate a greater openness to every form of psychotherapy, even though they adopt psychoanalysis as the frame of reference, but without submitting to the authority of a school: they know now that it can never substitute for the loss of the idea of the master. Whence a risk of eclecticism that can lead, if you don't watch out, to a dulling of theoretical rigor and, even more, to a forgetting of Freudian universalism.

This double rupture—first, with the ideal of the master and, second, with a single institutional model—seems irreversible. It is the mirror image of the splintering of the psychoanalytic field that can result in a positive reconfiguration of Freudian theory and clinical practice and in an acknowledgment of the new differences characteristic of modern subjectivity: exile, depression, self-victimization, discrimination on the part of the other, retreat into small communities, identity crisis, annihilation of thought, and so on.

In this connection, we can see why the two main concepts elaborated by Jacques Derrida—*difference* and *deconstruction*[7]—become so useful for many practitioners amid the current discontents of both psychoanalysis and society. The first enables them to think the idea of difference without yielding to differentialism, and the second enables them to give up the imperious figure of mastery but without effacing the Platonic ideal of the master.

Even in its failing, this ideal nonetheless remains the only one acting as an obstacle to the ravages of contemporary nihilism. So in the future, psychoanalysis should have to be able to remedy a real disaster, by weaving new links with philosophy, psychiatry, and the psychotherapies, thanks to the enthusiasm of the younger generations. And for this to happen it will again be necessary that it give a meaning to the conflicts that are bound to arise in the very heart of the depressive society.

Then the farcical image of behavior-modification man might well disappear, like a mirage dreamed up by the desert sands.

⊖

Notes

1. The Defeat of the Subject

1. On this topic, see Christophe Dejours, *Souffrance en France: La banalisation de l'injustice sociale* [Suffering in France: The becoming ordinary of social injustice] (Paris: Seuil, 1998).

2. This change was forecast ten years ago by Alain Renaut in *L'ère de l'individu* [The era of the individual] (Paris: Gallimard, 1989).

3. In the sense in which Georges Canguilhem uses this term in *La connaissance de la vie* [The knowledge of life] (Paris: Vrin, 1975).

4. I am here using the term *difference* in Jacques Derrida's sense. See chapter 11.

5. The discipline of psychopharmacology is dedicated to studying the effects of chemical substances on the brain.

6. For the history of cognitive science and the neurosciences, see chapter 5.

7. In a scathing work, *Les charlatans de la santé* [The health charlatans] (Paris: Payot, 1998), the psychiatrist Jean-Marie Abrall uses the word *patamedicine* for all these alternative medicines that claim to be substitutes for what is called scientific medicine by putting forward a "holistic" vision of illness, in other words taking into account its psychical dimension. The term *patamedicine* was invented by Marcel Francis Kahn.

8. See *L'Express*, January 30, 1997.

9. On this point, see Françoise Héritier's illuminating article "Les matrices de l'intolérance et de la violence" [The matrices of intolerance and violence], in *De la violence II* [Of violence II] (Paris: Odile Jacob, 1999), pp. 321–45.

10. See Viviane Forrester, *La violence du calme* [The violence of calm] (Paris: Seuil, 1980).

11. *Paradigm* is the term for the frame of thinking, the set of representations, or the specific model on the basis of which reflective thought is constructed during a given period. Each scientific revolution is translated through a change of paradigm. Nevertheless, in the field that concerns me here—medicine, psychiatry, and psychoanalysis—the coming of a new paradigm does not exclude that of the previous generation: it overlays it so as to give it a new meaning. See Thomas S. Kuhn, *The Structure of Scientific Revolutions* (Chicago: Chicago University Press, 1962).

12. Marcel Francis Kahn, "De notre mal, personne ne s'en rit" [No one is laughing at our hurt], in *Oedipe et les neurones* [Oedipus and neurones], *Autrement* 117 (October 1990): 171.

13. Marcel Gauchet has noted this phenomenon and is delighted that it makes it possible to announce the end of the omnipotence of the Freudian model. See "Essai de psychologie contemporaine, 1: Un nouvel âge de la personnalité" [Essay in contemporary psychology, 1: A new age of personality], *Le Débat* 100 (May–August 1998). The Canadian philosopher Charles Taylor also analyzes this phenomenon in *Sources of the Self: The Making of the Modern Identity* (Cambridge: Cambridge University Press, 1989).

14. Alain Ehrenberg, *La Fatigue d'être soi* [Tired of being oneself] (Paris: Odile Jacob, 1998), p. 17. Also note that Dr. Lowen-

stein, a specialist in drug addiction and director of the Monte-Christo Center at Laënnec hospital, has put forward the hypothesis of a structural link between high-level sport, depression, and addiction to a drug. "Why is it so hard for sportspeople to give up sport? Because it was fulfilling a role of antidepressive and anxiolytic bandage. There are so many things to be done: training, eating, taking vitamins. . . . When that is suppressed, sportspeople find themselves faced with the most painful thing: going back to thinking" (*Libération*, October 12, 1998).

2. The Medications of the Mind

1. See Jean Thuillier, *Les dix ans qui ont changé la folie* [The ten years that have changed madness] (Paris: Robert Laffont, 1981); Michel Reynaud and André Julien Coudert, *Essai sur l'art thérapeutique: Du bon usage des psychotropes* [An essay on therapeutic art: The correct use of psychotropic drugs] (Paris: Synapse–Frison Roche, 1987).

2. Jean Delay, "Allocution finale du colloque international sur la chlorpromazine et les médicaments neuroleptiques en psychiatrie" [Closing address at the international conference on chlorpromazine and neuroleptic medications in psychiatry], *L'Encéphale.* 45, no. 4 (1956): 1–81.

3. "Entretien avec Henri Laborit" [Interview with Henri Laborit], *Oedipe et les neurones* [Oedipus and neurones], *Autrement,* 117 (October 1990): 235.

4. Edouard Zarifian, *Des paradis plein la tête* [Head full of paradises] (1994; reprint, Paris: Odile Jacob, 1998), p. 73. A French psychiatrist, Zarifian denouces the excesses of psychopharmacology in *Le prix du bien-être: Psychotropes et société*

[The price of well-being: Psychotropic drugs and society] (Paris: Odile Jacob, 1996).

5. Put on the market in 1998 as the "happiness pill," first in the United States and then in the rest of the world, Viagra is a nonaphrodisiac vasodilator with no effect on sexual desire. It is only effective in relation to erectile dysfunctions linked to precise organic causes.

6. Zarifian, *Des paradis*, p. 32.

7. Michel Foucault gave the name "biopower" to a politics that claims to govern body and mind in the name of biology raised to the level of of a totalizing system and taking the place of religion. See Foucault, *"Il faut défendre la société": Cours au Collège de France, 1975–1976* ["Society must be defended": Collège de France seminars] (Paris: Seuil/Gallimard, 1997).

8. It is not said often enough that a common side effect of antidepressants is a lowering of sexual desire. With some men, they provoke manifestations of impotence.

9. Sigmund Freud and Josef Breuer, *Studies on Hysteria* (1895), in vol. 2 of *The Standard Edition of the Complete Psychological Works of Sigmund Freud*, trans. James Strachey (London: Hogarth, 1955–74).

10. See Ernest Jones, *The Life and Work of Sigmund Freud*, vol. 1, *1856–1900* (London: Hogarth, 1953); Henri F. Ellenberger, *The Discovery of the Unconscious: The History and Evolution of Dynamic Psychiatry* (New York: Basic, 1970); and *Médicines de l'âme: Essais d'histoire de la folie et des guérisons de l'âme* [Soul medicines: Essays in the history of madness and cures of the soul] (Paris: Fayard, 1995); Albrecht Hirschmüller, *The Life and Work of Josef Breuer: Physiology and Psychoanalysis* (New York: NYU Press, 1989).

11. Nosology is the discipline that studies the distinctive char-

acteristics of illnesses with a view to classification. Nosography is the discipline concerned with the classification and description of illnesses.

12. Patrick Froté, *Cent ans après* [A hundred years on] (interviews with Jean-Luc Donnet, André Green, Jean Laplanche, Jean-Claude Lavie, Joyce McDougall, Michel de M'Uzan, J.-B. Pontalis, Jean-Paul Valabrega, and Daniel Widlöcher) (Paris: Gallimard, 1998), p. 525. On the question of psychoanalytic institutions, see chapter 12.

13. Jacques Derrida, *Resistances of Psychoanalysis* (1996), trans. Peggy Kamuf, Pascale-Anne Brault, and Michael Naas (Stanford: Stanford University Press, 1998), p. 9.

14. Thus in the United States a new epidemic has been invented to designate hysteria: chronic fatigue syndrome. Linked to the notion of multiple personality (see chapter 3), this syndrome is treated with medication, and doctors say that it is caused by an as-yet-unidentified virus. See Elaine Showalter, *Hystories: Hysterical Epidemics and Modern Culture* (New York: Columbia University Press, 1997).

15. In France the consumption of tranquilizers and sleeping pills extends to 7 percent of the population, and that of antidepressants, constantly on the increase, 22 percent. In the United States psychostimulants are used in the same way as antidepressants in France. The consumption of neuroleptics (restricted to the psychoses) is stable in almost all countries, but it is set to increase slightly in the year 2000 with the appearance of new, more efficient molecules. See Marcel Legrain and Thérèse Lecomte, "La consommation des psychotropes en France et dans quelques pays européens" [The consumption of psychotropic drugs in France and in some other European countries], *Bulletin de l'Académie nationale de médecine* 181, no. 6 (1997): 1073–87. See

also Philippe Pignarre, *Puissance des psychotropes, pouvoir des patients* [Psychotropic drugs' capacity, patients' power] (Paris: PUF, 1999).

16. Pierre Juillet, "La société avant et depuis l'introduction des médicaments psychotropes en thérapeutique" [Society before and since the introduction of psychotropic medications in treatment], *Bulletin de l'Académie nationale de médecine* 181, no. 6 (1997): 1039–46.

17. See "Les médecins en état d'urgence: Boire toute l'angoisse des patients" [Doctors in a state of emergency: Drinking in all the patients' anguish], *Le Monde*, December 22, 1998.

3. The Soul Is Not a Thing

1. Pierre Jouve and Ali Magoudi, *Jacques Chirac: Portrait total* [Jacques Chirac: Total portrait] (Paris: Carrère, 1987); Georges Perec, *Penser/classer* [Thinking/classifying] (Paris: Hachette, 1995); Françoise Giroud: all quoted in *Le Nouvel Observateur*, September 14–20, 1995.

2. On this point, see H. J. Eysenck, "The Effects of Psychotherapy: An Evaluation," *Journal of Consultation and Psychology*, no. 16 (1952): 319–24; Clark Glymour, "Freud, Kepler, and the Clinical Evidence," in *Freud*, ed. Richard Wollheim (New York: Doubleday, Anchor, 1974), pp. 285–304; Bertrand Cramer, "Peut-on évaluer les effets des psychothérapies?" [Can the effects of psychotherapies be evaluated?], *Psychothérapies* 13, no. 4 (1993): 217–25; Adolf-Ernst Meyer, "Problèmes des études sur l'efficacité du processus psychothérapique" [Problems in studies of the effectiveness of the psychotherapeutic process], *Psychothérapies* 16, no. 2 (1996), 87–93; Daniel Widlöcher and

Alain Branconnier, eds., *Psychanalyse et psychothérapie* [Psychoanalysis and psychotherapy] (Paris: Flammarion, 1996). See also the opinion poll on French people's opinions of psychoanalysis conducted by *Le Nouvel Observateur* in 1980 (April 28–May 4).

3. Saul Rosenzweig, "An Experimental Study of Memory in Relation to the Theory of Repression," *British Journal of Psychology* 24 (1934): 247–65.

4. Fritz Wittels, *Freud and the Child Woman: The Memoirs of Fritz Wittels*, ed. Edward Timms (New Haven: Yale University Press, 1995), p. 150.

5. This is the method applied by two German-Swiss psychologists, Werner Greve and Jeanette Roos, in *Der Untergang des Ödipus-komplexes* [The decline of the Oedipus complex] (Berne: Hans Huber, 1996).

6. *Le Nouvel Observateur*, October 3–9, 1991, and September 14–20, 1995.

7. *Sciences et avenir*, February 1997. In particular, this report includes a long interview with Daniel Widlöcher, who praises Freud.

8. *Le Nouvel Observateur*, September 9–15, 1993, and March 20–26, 1997. One of these two issues is concerned with my 1993 book on Lacan (*Jacques Lacan: An Outline of a Life and a History of a System of Thought*, trans. Barbara Bray [New York: Columbia University Press, 1997]), the other with *Dictionnaire de la psychanalyse* [Dictionary of psychoanalysis], which I co-authored with Michel Plon (Paris: Fayard, 1997).

9. In an article on hypnosis in *Le Monde* of December 11, 1998, Véronique Maurus writes, on the subject of so-called short psychotherapies (which in fact have coexisted for half a century with psychoanalysis, their basic model): "Pragmatic and

measurable, they are gradually rendering outmoded the old kind of psychoanalysis, which today has practically been abandoned."

10. See Henri F. Ellenberger, *The Discovery of the Unconscious: The History and Evolution of Dynamic Psychiatry* (New York: Basic, 1970).

11. This is derived from the old psychology of peoples, according to which there exists for each nation, people, or race a specific mode of psychical organization. See part 3, chapter 3.

12. On the history of nineteenth-century psychiatry, see Jan Goldstein, *Console and Classify: The French Psychiatric Profession in the Nineteenth Century* (Cambridge: Cambridge University Press, 1987). Jacques Postel was the first to analyze the myth of the removal of the chains, in *Genèse de la psychiatrie: Les premiers écrits de Philippe Pinel* [The Genesis of Psychiatry: Early Writings of Philippe Pinel] (Le Plessis-Robinson: Synthélabo, 1998).

13. The idea that the division between humanity and animality overlays the difference between madness and reason is a constant in the history of psychiatry and madness. On this, see Elisabeth de Fontenay, *Le silence des bêtes* [The silence of the beasts] (Paris: Fayard, 1998).

4. Behavior-Modification Man

1. John Mann's article was published in the journal *Nature Médicine* in January 1998. See *Le Figaro*, February 11, 1998, where the protestations of Edouard Zarifian are also to be found. Serotonin is an excitatory chemical produced by intestinal and brain tissue that acts as a neurotransmitter. Some antidepressants (the SSRIs, or selective serotonin reuptake inhibitors) increase its

activity, whence the idea that depression might be due simply to a lowering of serotonin activity.

2. On this question, see Elisabeth Roudinesco and Michel Plon, *Dictionnaire de la psychanalyse* [Dictionary of psycho-analysis] (Paris: Fayard, 1997), s.v. "Suicide." And on the ancient and modern figures of suicidology, see Maurice Pinguet, *La mort volontaire au Japon* [Voluntary death in Japan] (Paris: Gallimard, 1984).

3. Interview with Steven Rose, *Libération*, March 21, 1995.

4. On the critique of this position, see chapter 11.

5. On this question, see Fethi Benslama, "Qu'est-ce qu'une clinique de l'exil?" [What is a treatment for exile?], *Cahiers Intersignes*, 14 (1999).

6. Sigmund Freud, *An Outline of Psycho-Analysis* (1940), in *The Standard Edition of the Complete Psychological Works of Sigmund Freud*, trans. James Strachey (London: Hogarth, 1955–74), 23:182.

7. Gladys Swain, "Chimie, cerveau, esprit et société" [Chemistry, brain, mind, and society] (1987), in *Dialogue avec l'insensé* [Dialogue with the senseless] (Paris: Gallimard, 1994), p. 269.

8. See Stuart Kirk and Herb Kutchins, *The Selling of DSM: The Rhetoric of Science in Psychiatry* (New York: Walter de Gruyter, 1992).

9. Georges Canguilhem has some magnificent pages on this subject in *The Normal and the Pathological* (1943) (New York: Zone, 1989).

10. Edouard Zarifian has described this drift extremely well in *Des paradis plein la tête* [Head full of paradises] (1994; reprint, Paris: Odile Jacob, 1998).

11. Quoted in Kirk and Kutchins, *The Selling*.

12. Quoted in ibid.

5. Frankenstein's Brain

1. Georges Canguilhem, "Le cerveau et la pensée" (1980) [The brain and thought], in *Georges Canguilhem: Philosophe, historien des sciences* [Georges Canguilhem: Philosopher, historian of science] (Paris: Albin Michel, 1992), pp. 11–33; "Qu'est-ce que la psychologie?" [What is psychology?] (1956), in *Etudes d'histoire de la philosophie des sciences* [Studies in the history of the philosophy of science] (Paris: Vrin, 1968). On the earlier text, see Elisabeth Roudinesco, "Situation d'un texte: Qu'est-ce que la psychologie?" [Situating a text: "What is psychology?"] in *Georges Canguilhem*, pp. 135–44.

2. This is how Canguilhem characterized psychology in 1956.

3. Canguilhem, "Le cerveau," p. 17. Invented by Franz-Josef Gall (1748–1818), the so-called science of cerebral localizations (or craniology) claimed to explain an individual's character through the study of the projections and hollows of the cranium. It was Thomas Forster, an English disciple of Gall's, who invented the term *phrenology*.

4. John R. Searle criticized the supporters of this thesis as severely as Canguilhem in *Minds, Brains, and Science* (Cambridge: Harvard University Press, 1985).

5. Claude Bernard, *Introduction à l'étude de la médicine expérimentale* [Introduction to the study of experimental medicine] (Paris: Baillière, 1865), p. 9.

6. There can be no doubt that at this time Georges Canguilhem had carefully read Foucault's *Madness and Civilization* and *Discipline and Punish*. And after the philosopher's death, he was to stress the extent to which Foucault was seeking the explanation of certain practices in forms of power, where strenuous efforts had been made to find the backup for those practices in sci-

ence. See Michel Foucault, *Madness and Civilization: A History of Insanity in the Age of Reason* (1961), trans. Richard Howard (1967; reprint, London: Routledge, 1999); *Discipline and Punish: The Birth of the Prison* (1975), trans. Alan Sheridan (1977; reprint, New York: Vintage, 1979); Georges Canguilhem, "Sur l'*Histoire de la folie* comme événement" [On *Madness and Civilization* as an event], *Le Débat*, no. 41 (1986).

7. On this see Monique Vacquin, *Frankenstein; ou, Les délires de la raison* [Frankenstein; or, Reason's madness] (Paris: François Bourin, 1990); Dominique Lecourt, *Prométhée, Faust, Frankenstein: Fondements imaginaires de l'éthique* [Prometheus, Faust, Frankenstein: Imaginary foundations of ethics] (1996; reprint, Paris: Livre de Poche, "Biblio-Essais," 1998).

8. On this, see François Bouyssi, *Alfred Giard et ses élèves: Un cénacle de philosophes biologistes: Aux origines du scientisme?* [Alfred Giard and his pupils: An inner circle of biologist philosophers: The starting point of the origins of scientism?], EPHE [Ecole Polytechnique des Hautes Etudes] thesis supervised by Pierre Legendre, Paris, 1998.

9. Sigmund Freud, *The Future of an Illusion* (1927), in *The Standard Edition of the Complete Psychological Works of Sigmund Freud*, trans. James Strachey (London: Hogarth, 1955–74), 21:5–56.

10. Henri Korn, "L'inconscient à l'épreuve des neurosciences" [The unconscious tested by the neurosciences], *Le Monde diplomatique*, September 1989, 1.

11. Jean-Pierre Changeux, *L'homme neuronal* [Neuronal man] (Paris: Fayard, 1983); and "Entretien" [Interview], in *Le Courrier du CNRS*, April–June 1984, pp. 5–11.

12. Marcel Gauchet, *L'inconscient cérébral* [The cerebral unconscious] (Paris: Seuil, 1992), p. 182.

13. Francis Fukuyama, "La fin de l'histoire, dix ans après" [The end of history, ten years later], *Le Monde*, June 17, 1999.

14. Gerald M. Edelman, *The Remembered Present: A Biological Theory of Consciousness* (New York: Basic, 1989).

15. *Le Nouvel Observateur*, March 20–26, 1997, p. 14. The neurophysiologist Jean-Didier Vincent takes up an identical position in *Biologie des passions* (Paris: Odile Jacob/Seuil, 1986). See also Bernard Andrieu, *L'homme naturel: La fin promise des sciences humaines* [Natural man: The promised end of the sciences] (Lyon: Presses universitaires de Lyon, 1999).

16. Sigmund Freud, *Project for a Scientific Psychology* (1895), in *Standard Edition*, 1:294–397.

17. Henri F. Ellenberger, *The Discovery of the Unconscious: The History and Evolution of Dynamic Psychiatry* (New York: Basic, 1970), p. 507.

18. Sigmund Freud, "The Unconscious" (1915), in *Standard Edition*, 14:174; idem, *Beyond the Pleasure Principle* (1920), in *Standard Edition*, 18:60.

19. Frank J. Sulloway offered an impressive analysis of the different readings that have been given of the *Project* in *Freud, Biologist of the Mind: Beyond the Psychoanalytic Legend* (New York: Basic, 1979).

20. The first use of the term in a conceptual sense was in 1751: the evidence is a text in English. It was then popularized in Germany and introduced in France around 1860. See Elisabeth Roudinesco and Michel Plon, *Dictionnaire de la psychanalyse* [Dictionary of psychoanalysis] (Paris: Fayard, 1997); and Lancelot Law Whyte, *The Unconscious Before Freud* (1960; reprint, New York: Basic, 1962).

21. This question has been debated at length by Michel Foucault and Jacques Derrida. See Foucault, *Madness and Civiliza-*

tion; and Jacques Derrida, "Cogito and the History of Madness" (1964), in *Writing and Difference* (1967), trans. Alan Bass (Chicago: University of Chicago Press, 1977).

22. Michel Foucault, *The Will to Knowledge: A History of Sexuality,* Vol. *1* (1976), trans. Robert Hurley (1978; reprint, London: Penguin, 1998). I studied this configuration of heredity-degeneration myself in *La bataille de cent ans: Historie de la psychanalyse en France* [The hundred-year battle: A history of psychoanalysis in France], vol. 1, *1885–1939* (1982; reprint, Paris: Fayard, 1994). See also Zeev Sternhell, *La droite révolutionnaire* [The revolutionary right] (Paris: Seuil, 1978).

23. It is this cerebral unconscious that Marcel Gauchet wants to put in the place of the Freudian unconscious. See Gauchet, *L'inconscient cérébral.*

24. See Roudinesco and Plon, *Dictionnaire*; and Ellenberger, *The Discovery.* For Herbart's influence, see Ola Andersson, *Studies in the Prehistory of Psychoanalysis* (Upsala: Norstedts, 1997).

25. As Michel Jouvet stresses in *Le sommeil et le rêve* [Sleep and dreaming] (Paris: Odile Jacob, 1992).

6. The "Equinox Letter"

1. Sigmund Freud, "A Difficulty in the Path of Psycho-analysis" (1917), in *The Standard Edition of the Complete Psychological Works of Sigmund Freud,* trans. James Strachey (London: Hogarth, 1955–74), 17:143.

2. Frank J. Sulloway has highlighted the theories from which Freud took his inspiration. Nonetheless, I do not share that author's idea that Freud remained a "biologist of the mind." On this, see Michel Plon's preface to the French translation of

Sulloway's book (chapter 5, note 21), *Freud, biologiste de l'esprit* (Paris: Fayard, 1998).

3. *The Complete Letters of Sigmund Freud to Wilhelm Fliess, 1887–1904*, trans. and ed. Jeffrey Moussaieff Masson (Cambridge: Harvard University Press, Belknap, 1985), pp. 264, 266.

4. See ibid.

5. This riposte from Freud, who considered the dogma of sexual theory as a "bulwark" against occultism, was reported by Carl Gustav Jung, *Memories, Dreams, Reflections*, trans. Richard Winston and Clara Winston (1963; reprint, London: Fontana, 1995), p. 173.

6. *The Complete Correspondence of Sigmund Freud and Ernest Jones, 1908–1939*, ed. R. Andrew Paskauskas, trans. Riccardo Steiner (Cambridge: Harvard University Press, Belknap, 1993).

7. Michel Foucault, "La recherche scientifique et la psychologie" [Scientific research and psychology] (1957), in *Dits et écrits* [Spoken and written words], vol. 1 (Paris: Gallimard, 1994), pp. 153–54.

8. Jean Delumeau and Daniel Roche, eds., *Histoire des pères et de la paternité* [A history of fathers and paternity] (Paris: Larousse, 1990).

9. Michel Foucault also thinks that psychoanalysis was the instrument of a new control over incestuous relations in the middle-class family. See *Les anormaux: Cours au Collège de France, 1974–5* [The abnormal: Collège de France seminars, 1974–5] (Paris: Gallimard/Seuil, 1999).

10. On the family as a universal model, see chapter 9.

11. See further the great American psychoanalyst Leonard Shengold's fine book, *Soul Murder: The Effects of Childhood Abuse and Deprivation* (New Haven: Yale University Press,

1989). See, too, Boris Cyrulnik, *Un merveilleux malheur* [A wonderful misfortune] (Paris: Odile Jacob, 1999).

12. It should be noted that the Kleinians, without denying the existence of actual abuse, tended to think that imaginary seductions of a sadistic kind could be much more serious than actual traumas. Sandor Ferenczi and his heirs, on the other hand, gave the place of honor back to the idea of the importance of the lived trauma, against the orthodoxies of fantasy.

13. The theme of pansymbolism was widely exploited in France in the first half of the century. See Elisabeth Roudinesco, *La bataille de cent ans: Historie de la psychanalyse en France* [The hundred-year battle: A history of psychoanalysis in France] (1982; reprint, Paris: Fayard, 1994).

7. Freud Is Dead in America

1. See François Eustache, "L'inconscient cognitif: Chronique d'un concept" [The cognitive unconscious: Story of a concept], in *Le corps et le sens* [The body and meaning], ed. Bianca Lechevalier and Bernard Lechevalier (Lausanne: Delachaux and Niestlé, 1998), pp. 247–75.

2. Howard Gardner, *The Mind's New Science: A History of the Cognitive Revolution* (New York: Basic, 1985). It is worth noting that Jean Piaget (1896–1980), pioneer of cognitive psychology, was only interested in the universal character of mental development and of the evolution of intellectual capacities.

3. Behaviorism is a strand of psychology that flourished in the United States up to 1950 and until it collapsed constituted a serious barrier to the reception of psychoanalysis in that country. It is based on the idea that human behavior obeys the

principle of stimulus-response (SR). It is thus a variant of behavior-modification therapy, whereas so-called cognitive psychology assumes further a modeling of internal psychical activity. Still, behaviorism is often classified as part of cognitive psychology, whence a certain confusion in the way that the different strands are grasped.

4. Gardner, *The Mind's New Science*, p. 15.

5. See Michel Plon, *La théorie des jeux: Une politique imaginaire* [Game theory: An imaginary politics] (Paris: Maspero, 1976).

6. Gerald M. Edelman, *The Remembered Present: A Biological Theory of Consciousness* (New York: Basic, 1989). See also Francisco Varela, *Connaître: Les sciences cognitives: Tendances et perspectives* [Knowing: The cognitive sciences: Tendencies and perspectives] (Paris: Seuil, 1989); and Daniel Andler, ed., *Introduction aux sciences cognitives* [Introduction to the cognitive sciences], (Paris: Gallimard, Folio, 1992). Varela comes over as very critical toward the trends in cognitivism against which he sets up his own conception of cognition (not very different, however, from the ones he rejects). It is worth pointing out that André Green has written an extremely good study of these divergences and made clear the aporias of cognitivism, though I cannot follow him when he aligns Lacan's work on the side of cognitive science by making structuralism the equivalent of a logistical theory that gets rid of subjectivity (in *La causalité psychique* [Psychical causality] [Paris: Odile Jacob, 1994]). For identical reasons, it is hard to subscribe to the positions of Daniel Widlöcher, who, contrary to André Green, maintains in *Les nouvelles cartes de la psychanalyse* [The new maps of psychoanalysis] (Paris: Odile Jacob, 1996) that cognitive science and the Freudian theory of the unconscious are compatible.

7. Lawrence A. Hirschfeld, "The One-Drop-of-Blood Rule; or, How the Child Acquires the Idea of Race" (1996), published in French in *L'Homme*, no. 150 (April–June 1999); idem, *Race in the Making: Cognition, Culture, and the Child's Construction of Human Kinds* (Cambridge, Mass.: MIT Press, 1996).

8. It was through an official declaration that UNESCO effectively let go of this notion, stressing the fundamental unity of the human species and rejecting biological differences as epiphenomena. Claude Lévi-Strauss was among the signatories: see *Race and History* (Paris: UNESCO, 1952).

9. Published in 1933, the novel was adapted in 1959 by Douglas Sirk, who transformed it wholesale to make it into a sumptuous Hollywood melodrama.

10. Howard Gardner, *Extraordinary Minds: Portraits of Exceptional Individuals and an Examination of Extraordinariness* (1997; reprint, London: Phoenix, 1998).

11. Christopher D. Frith, *The Cognitive Neuropsychology of Schizophrenia* (Hove: Lawrence Erlbaum, 1992). See also Patricia Smith Churchland, *Neurophilosophy: Toward a Unified Science of the Mind-Brain* (Cambridge, Mass.: MIT Press, 1985); and Henri Grivois and Joëlle Proust, eds., *Subjectivité et conscience d'agir: Approches cognitives et cliniques de la psychose* [Subjectivity and consciousness of action: Cognitive and clinical approaches to psychosis] (Paris: PUF, 1998).

12. From Frank Buchman, founder of Moral Rearmament, a sectarian movement whose aim is the "regeneration of humanity."

13. Wittels, *Freud*, pp. 148–49.

14. See Nathan G. Hale Jr., *Freud in America*, vol. 1, *Freud and the Americans: The Beginnings of Psychoanalysis in the United States, 1876–1917* (New York: Oxford University Press, 1971), and vol. 2, *The Rise and Crisis of Psychoanalysis in the*

United States: Freud and the Americans, 1917–1985 (Oxford: Oxford University Press, 1995); and idem, ed., *James Jackson Putnam and Psychoanalysis: Letters Between Putnam and Sigmund Freud, Ernest Jones, William James, Sandor Ferenczi, and Morton Prince, 1877–1917* (Cambridge: Harvard University Press, 1971).

15. Freud to Wittels, letters of July 11 and August 7, 1928, in Wittels, *Freud*, p. 130.

16. Adolf Grünbaum, *The Foundations of Psychoanalysis: A Philosophical Critique* (Berkeley: University of California Press, 1984). In a later piece, entitled "Is Freud's Theory Well-Founded?" (*Behavioral and Brain Sciences* 9, no. 2 [1986]: 266–81), Grünbaum responded to his critics.

17. Karl Popper, *Conjectures and Refutations: The Growth of Scientific Knowledge* (1963), 5th ed. (New York: Routledge, 1989); idem, *Realism and the Aim of Science* (London: Hutchinson, 1983); Paul Ricoeur, *Freud and Philosophy: An Essay on Interpretation* (1965), trans. Denis Savage (New Haven: Yale University Press, 1970); Jürgen Habermas, *Knowledge and Human Interests* (1968), trans. Jeremy J. Shapiro (Boston: Beacon, 1971).

18. On this question, see chapter 9.

19. See chapter 3.

20. Sigmund Freud, "Notes Upon a Case of Obsessional Neurosis" (1909), in *The Standard Edition of the Complete Psychological Works of Sigmund Freud*, trans. James Strachey (London: Hogarth, 1955–74), 10:153–318.

21. Sigmund Freud, "From the History of an Infantile Neurosis" (1918), in *Standard Edition*, 17:3–122; Muriel Gardiner, ed., *The Wolf Man by the Wolf Man* (New York: Basic, 1971); Karin Obholzer, *The Wolf-Man: Conversations with Freud's Patient—*

Sixty Years Later (1980), trans. Michael Shaw (New York: Continuum, 1982). On the different interpretations of the two case histories, see Elisabeth Roudinesco and Michel Plon, *Dictionnaire de la psychanalyse* [Dictionary of psychoanalysis] (Paris: Fayard, 1997).

22. Marie Bonaparte, *Cinq cahiers écrits par une petite fille entre sept ans et demi et dix ans, avec leurs commentaires* [Five notebooks written by a little girl between the ages of seven and a half and ten, with commentaries], 4 vols. (published by the author, 1939–51); idem, "Extraits du Cahier I" [Extracts from notebook I], *L'Infini*, no. 2 (spring 1983): 76–89.

23. See "La science contre la psychanalyse" [Science against psychoanalysis], *Le Nouvel Observateur*, November 1–7, 1990, p. 27.

24. J. M. Masson, *The Assault on Truth: Freud's Suppression of the Seduction Theory* (New York: Farrar, Strauss, and Giroux, 1984). See, too, Janet Malcolm, *In the Freud Archives* (London: Jonathan Cape, 1984).

25. The term *revisionism* was adopted by a certain number of U.S. researchers demanding a revision of the founding concepts of Freudian theory. This trend has nothing to do with the negationism that denies the existence of the gas chambers.

26. Catherine MacKinnon, *Feminism Unmodified: Discourses on Life and Law* (Cambridge: Harvard University Press, 1987); Judith Herman, *Trauma and Recovery* (New York: Basic, 1992).

27. See Henri F. Ellenberger, *The Discovery of the Unconscious: The History and Evolution of Dynamic Psychiatry* (New York: Basic, 1970).

28. In his book *Rewriting the Soul: Multiple Personality and the Sciences of Memory* (Princeton: Princeton University Press,

1995), Ian Hacking has described this phenomenon. But he attributes its causes to the American obsession with child sexual abuse, not to the anti-Freud crusade.

29. Frank J. Sulloway, *Biologist of the Mind: Beyond the Psychoanalytic Legend* (New York: Basic, 1979).

30. In the United States, Paul Robinson pointed out these excesses extremely well in *Freud and His Critics* (Berkeley: University of California Press, 1993).

31. See Michelle Le Barzic and Marianne Pouillon, *La meilleure façon de manger* [The best way to eat] (Paris: Odile Jacob, 1998).

32. See Frédéric Filloux, "Echec aux manipulateurs du souvenir en Californie" [Memory manipulators in California lose case], *Libération*, May 17, 1994, p. 20.

33. This unbelievable story is told by Stuart A. Kirk and Herb Kutchins in *The Selling of DSM: The Rhetoric of Science in Psychiatry* (New York: Walter de Gruyter, 1992).

8. A French Scientism

1. Louis Althusser, *Ecrits sur la psychanalyse* [Writings on psychoanalysis] (Paris: Stock-IMEC, 1993).

2. See Elisabeth Roudinesco, *La bataille de cent ans: Historie de la psychanalyse en France* [The hundred-year battle: A history of psychoanalysis in France] (1982; reprint, Paris: Fayard, 1994); and Serge Moscovici, *La psychanalyse, son image et son public* [Psychoanalysis, its image and its public] (Paris: PUF, 1976).

3. Pierre Debray-Ritzen, *La scolastique freudienne* [Freudian scholasticism] (Paris: Fayard, 1972).

4. Jean-Pierre Changeux and Paul Ricoeur, *La nature et la règle* [Nature and rules] (Paris: Seuil, 1998), p. 240. See, too, Dominique Lecourt, *L'Amérique entre la Bible et Darwin* [America between the Bible and Darwin] (Paris: PUF, 1992).

5. The term was proposed by Jacques Derrida.

6. I developed this idea in *Généalogies* [Genealogies] (Paris: Fayard, 1994).

7. Hannah Arendt, *On Revolution* (1963), 2d ed. (New York: Viking, 1965).

8. We recall Robespierre's famous prophecy: "We shall perish because in the history of humanity we have not been able to find the moment to found Liberty."

9. Science and Psychoanalysis

1. Typed document of July 31, 1995.

2. This petition, which I wrote myself with Philippe Garnier, was published in *Les Carnets de psychanalyse*, no. 8 (1997). On the surrounding polemics, see *Le Monde*, June 14, 1996.

3. Interview with Patrick Sabatier, *Libération*, October 26, 1998.

4. Michael Roth, ed., *Freud, Conflict, and Culture: Essays on His Life, Work, and Legacy* (New York: Knopf, 1998).

5. Relativism is a critical attitude that consists of systematically challenging all established truths, including the most irrefutable facts, so as to counter them with the idea that all truths are constructed according to a dominant culture. This trend is close to revisionism and derives—pushing them to absurdity—from critical and deconstructive theses coming from philosophy, anthropology, and psychoanalysis.

6. Alan Sokal and Jean Bricmont, *Impostures intellectuelles* (Paris: Odile Jacob, 1997). [The English version, *Intellectual Impostures: Postmodern Philosophers' Abuse of Science* (London: Profile Books, 1998), has apparently been revised in light of some of the criticisms made by Roudinesco, recapitulated in the present volume, when the French edition first appeared. See Elisabeth Roudinesco, "Sokal et Bricmont sont-ils des imposteurs?" [Are Sokal and Bricmont impostors?], *L'Infini* 62 (summer 1998): 19–21. —Trans.]

7. Richard Macksey and Eugenio Donato, *The Structuralist Controversy: The Languages of Criticism and the Sciences of Man* (Baltimore: Johns Hopkins University Press, 1970), pp. 186–95.

8. Sokal and Bricmont, *Impostures*, p. 17.

9. In Jacques Lacan, *Ecrits* (Paris: Seuil, 1966), pp. 855–77.

10. Jacques Lacan, *Le séminaire, livre VI, 1958–1959: Le désir et son interprétation* [Desire and its interpretation], unpublished.

11. Nowadays we readily speak of the social sciences to designate the human sciences and so distinguish the sciences of humanity, which include the dimension of subjectivity, from those that exclude it. The sciences can also be divided into two branches: sciences of nature and sciences of culture. See Max Weber, *The Methodology of the Social Sciences*, trans. and ed. Edward A. Shils and Henry A. Finch (New York: Free, 1949).

12. Gilles Gaston Granger, *L'Irrationnel* [The irrational] (Paris: Odile Jacob, 1998).

13. A term invented in 1882 by the English psychologist Frederick Myers (1843–1901) to designate a long-range communication by thought (or transmission of thought) between two persons thought to be in a psychical relationship.

14. See Rony Brauman and Eyal Sival's film *Le Spécialiste* [The specialist].

15. Hannah Arendt, *Eichmann in Jerusalem* (New York: Viking, 1963).

16. See, too, Lacan, "Kant avec Sade" [Kant with Sade] (1963), in *Ecrits*, pp. 765–90.

17. Claude Lanzmann, in *L'Evénement*, April 8–14, 1999, p. 92.

18. See Raul Hilberg, *The Destruction of the European Jews* (New York: Holmes, 1985).

19. Sigmund Freud, *Civilization and Its Discontents* (1930), in *The Standard Edition of the Complete Psychological Works of Sigmund Freud*, trans. James Strachey (London: Hogarth, 1955–74), 21:145.

20. Texts by Freud on telepathy and occultism include "Psychoanalysis and Telepathy" (1921) and "Dreams and Telepathy" (1922), *Standard Edition*, 18:175–193, 197–220; and "Dreams and Occultism" (1933), *Standard Edition*, 22:31–56. See also Wladimir Granoff and Jean-Michel Rey, *L'occulte, objet de la pensée freudienne* [The occult, object of Freudian thought] (Paris: PUF, 1983). The best commentary is Jacques Derrida's: "Telepathy" (1981), trans. Nicholas Royle, *Oxford Literary Review* 10 (1988): 3–41.

21. The concept of deconstruction was introduced by Jacques Derrida. See chapter 12.

22. Freud, *The Psychopathology of Everyday Life* (1905), in *Standard Edition*, 6:259.

10. Tragic Man

1. Jean Starobinski, "Hamlet et Freud," in Ernest Jones, *Hamlet et Oédipe* (Paris: Gallimard, 1967). [Starobinski's essay

does not appear in the original English version, *Hamlet and Freud* (London: Victor Gollancz, 1949).—Trans.]

2. Karl Popper, *Conjectures and Refutations: The Growth of Scientific Knowledge* (1963), 5th ed. (New York: Routledge, 1989). Popper lumps psychoanalysis together with the Marxist theory of history and Alfred Adler's individual psychology.

3. In Elisabeth Roudinesco and Michel Plon, *Dictionnaire de la psychanalyse* [Dictionary of psychoanalysis] (Paris: Fayard, 1997), we counted six large schools: Anna-Freudianism, Kleinianism, ego psychology, the Independent Group, self psychology, and Lacanianism.

4. See Eugène Enriquez, *De la horde à l'Etat* [From horde to state] (Paris: Gallimard, 1983).

5. See Carl Schorske, *Fin-de-siècle Vienna: Politics and Culture* (London: Weidenfeld and Nicholson, 1980).

6. Winnicott speaks in this connection of a "false self," in "Distortion of the Self in Relation to True and False Selves," in *The Maturational Processes and the Facilitating Environment* (London: Hogarth, 1965). In psychoanalytic terminology, the ego is an aspect of the psyche deriving from the unconscious, whereas the self is an imaginary representation of oneself for oneself. In phenomenological terms, it is an aspect of the personality that is set up later than the ego.

7. The imago is an unconscious representation enabling the subject to construct for him- or herself an image of her relations with her parents.

8. Claude Lévi-Strauss, *The Elementary Structures of Kinship* (1949), trans. James Harle Bell and John Richardson Sturmer, ed. Rodney Needham (Boston: Beacon, 1969).

9. This term, through which Lacan defines the signifier of the paternal function, appeared for the first time as a concept in

1956, in *Le séminaire, livre III: Les psychoses (1955–1956)* [The seminar, book III: The psychoses (1955–1956)] (Paris: Seuil, 1981). See Elisabeth Roudinesco, *Jacques Lacan: An Outline of a Life and a History of a System of Thought*, trans. Barbara Bray (New York: Columbia University Press, 1997); and Erik Porge, *Les noms du père chez Lacan* [The names of the father in Lacan] (Toulouse: Erès, 1997).

10. Theodor W. Adorno and Max Horkheimer, *Dialectic of Enlightenment* (1944), trans. John Cumming (New York: Seabury, Continuum, 1972).

11. Claude Lévi-Strauss, "La famille" (The family) (1956), in *Textes de et sur Claude Levi-Strauss*, ed. Raymond Bellour and Catherine Clement (Paris: Gallimard, Idées, 1975), p. 95.

12. Jacques Lacan, *Le séminaire, livre IV: La relation d'objet (1956–1957)* [Seminars, book IV: The object relation (1956–1957)] (Paris: Seuil, 1994), pp. 375–76. On this question, see the discussion between Robert Badinter and Françoise Héritier, *Masculin/féminin: La pensée de la différence* [Masculine/feminine: The thinking of difference] (Paris: Odile Jacob, 1996).

13. Some practitioners however have courageously approached the problem, especially Geneviève Delaisi de Parceval, who wrote a preface to Eric Dubreuil's book, *Des parents du même sexe* [Parents of the same sex] (Paris: Odile Jacob, 1998).

14. On this topic, see Michel Foucault, *Les anormaux: Cours de Collège de France (1974–1975)* [The abnormal: Collège de France seminars, 1974–1975], ed. Valerio Marchetti and Antonella Salomoni, Hautes Etudes series (Paris: Gallimard/Seuil, 1999).

15. [Baron Charlus is a homosexual character in Proust's *A la recherche du temps perdu.—*Trans.]

11. Universality, Difference, Exclusion

1. See Elisabeth Roudinesco, *Généalogies* [Genealogies] (Paris: Fayard, 1994).

2. In a lecture given in March 1999, Alain Finkielkraut summarized this situation with a striking formulation: "I suffer, therefore I accuse." See, too, Eugène Enriquez, "Tuer sans culpabilité" [Killing without guilt], *L'Inactuel*, no. 2 (spring 1999): 15–36.

3. On this, see André Kaspi, *Mal connus, mal aimés, mal compris: les Etats-Unis d'aujourd'hui* [Little known, little loved, misunderstood: The United States today] (Paris: Plon, 1999).

4. See Sélim Abou, "L'universel et la relativité des cultures" [The universal and the relativity of cultures], in *L'Idée d'humanité* [The idea of humanity] (Paris: Albin Michel, 1995); and John. R. Searle, "Is There a Crisis in American Higher Education?" *Partisan Review* 60, no. 4 (1993): 693–709.

5. The effects of this were apparent in February 1999 when the French parliament voted in a law registering the difference of the sexes in article 3 of the constitution.

6. See Wiktor Stoczkowski's article "La pensée de l'exclusion et la pensée de la différence" [The thinking of exclusion and the thinking of difference], *L'Homme*, no. 150 (April–June 1999): 41–57. The author shows how racism feeds on ambivalences between a rigid notion of exclusion and just as rigid a notion of difference.

7. Sigmund Freud, *The Future of an Illusion* (1927), *The Standard Edition of the Complete Psychological Works of Sigmund Freud*, trans. James Strachey (London: Hogarth, 1955–74), 21:7.

12. Critique of Psychoanalytic Institutions

1. [The Haskalah was an eighteenth- and nineteenth-century movement, originating in Germany, to make Jews and Judaism more cosmopolitan. It encouraged interest in non-Jewish art and thought and the adoption of local ways—clothes, customs, language.—Trans.]

2. I put forward this idea in 1982 in *La bataille de cent ans: Historie de la psychanalyse en France* [The hundred-year battle: A history of psychoanalysis in France] (1982; reprint, Paris: Fayard, 1994), vol. 1.

3. Lay analysis is analysis practiced by those who are not medical doctors.

4. See Roudinesco, *La bataille*, vols. 1 and 2; idem, *Jacques Lacan and Co.: A History of Psychoanalysis in France, 1925–1985* (1986), trans. Jeffrey Mehlman (Chicago: University of Chicago Press, 1990); and idem, *Jacques Lacan: An Outline of a Life and a History of a System of Thought*, trans. Barbara Bray (New York: Columbia University Press, 1997).

5. Jacques Lacan, "Proposition du 9 octobre 1967 sur le psychanalyste de l'Ecole" [Proposition of October 9, 1967, on the School psychoanalyst], *Scilicet* 1 (1968): 14–30; first version in *Analytica* 8, supplement to *Ornicar?* (1978): 15.

6. [The formulation *être-analyste* also implies, more philosophically and more grandly, *analyst-being*.—Trans.]

7. Jacques Derrida writes *differance*, with an *a*, to indicate that difference is not a division between two states or two kinds, neither a presence nor an absence, but a movement inscribed on the One, on which it imprints a detour, a division, an inequality, a displacement. See Jacques Derrida, *Writing and Difference* (1967), trans. Alan Bass (Chicago: University of Chicago Press, 1978).

Index

EUROPEAN PERSPECTIVES

A Series in Social Thought and Cultural Criticism

Lawrence D. Kritzman, Editor

EUROPEAN PERSPECTIVES presents outstanding books by leading European thinkers. With both classic and contemporary works, the series aims to shape the major intellectual controversies of our day and to facilitate the tasks of historical understanding.